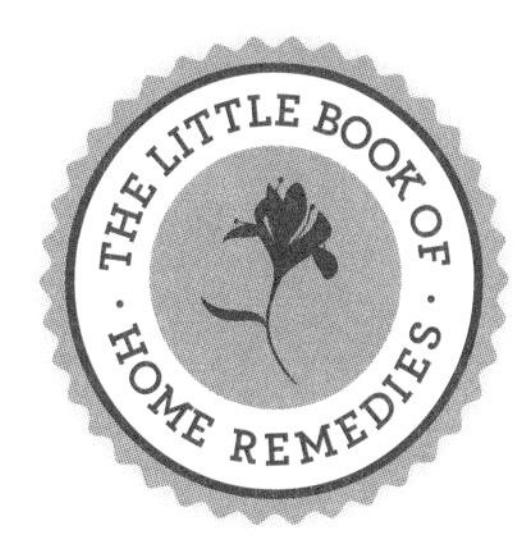

BEAUTY
— *and* —
HEALTH

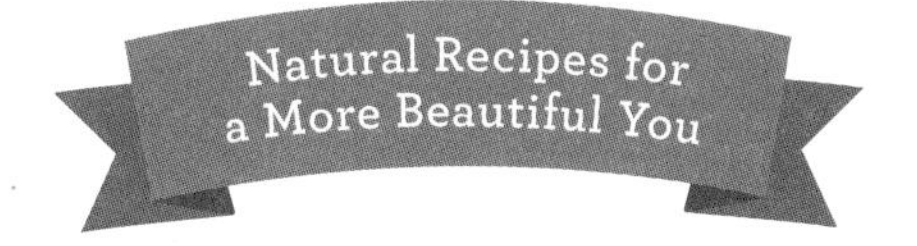

Linda B. White, M.D.
Barbara H. Seeber & Barbara Brownell Grogan

First published in the USA in 2015 by
Fair Winds Press, a member of
Quarto Publishing Group USA Inc.
100 Cummings Center
Suite 406-L
Beverly, MA 01915-6101
www.fairwindspress.com
Visit www.bodymindbeautyhealth.com. It's your personal guide to a happy, healthy, and extraordinary life!

19 18 17 16 15 1 2 3 4 5

ISBN: 978-1-59233-671-5

Content for this book was previously published in the book *500 Time-Tested Home Remedies and the Science Behind Them* by Linda B. White, M.D., Barbara Brownell Grogan, and Barbara H. Seeber (Fair Winds Press, 2014).

Cover design by Leigh Ring // RingArtDesign.com
Book design by Leigh Ring // RingArtDesign.com

The information in this book is for educational purposes only. It is not intended to replace the advice of a physician or medical practitioner. Please see your health care provider before beginning any new health program. The authors and publisher are not responsible for readers' misuse of these recipes and, as a result, any unintended effects.

Printed and bound in USA

Contents

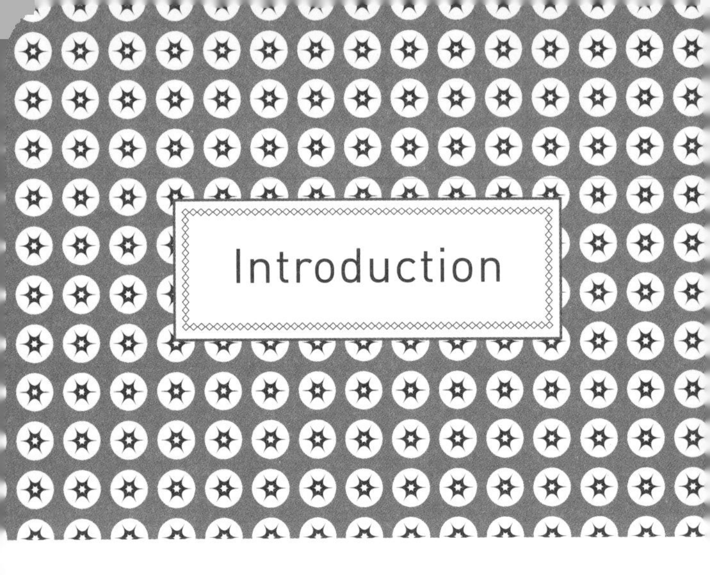

Introduction

In today's high-powered, health-conscious world, we're all smarter, more informed about our bodies, and preoccupied with ways to live long, healthy lives. We've accomplished half of that goal: living longer. But we're missing the "living healthier" part of the equation.

On December 15, 2012, the British medical journal *The Lancet* published data from the Global Burden of Disease Study 2010. Here are the key findings, starting with the good news: Around the world, longevity has increased. We're less likely to succumb prematurely to malaria and measles, but more likely to drop dead later in life from heart attack or stroke. The bad news is, we're more likely to spend our last years disabled by diseases—most of which are preventable.

Chronic illness has long dogged Americans. Now it's spreading to other countries. Where have we gone wrong? We have health-related facts and figures at our fingertips. We have expensive diagnostic tests, highly trained doctors, and cutting-edge treatments. The shelves in supermarkets groan under the weight of boxes, cans, and bags. Modern conveniences have reduced our need for physical labor. Computers give us up-to-date medical bulletins.

Despite these advances, and to some extent because of them, we've become fat, flabby, and frequently ill. We're too often hurried, harried, sleep-deprived, and socially disconnected. We eat in our cars, at our desks, in front of televisions—everywhere but at the dining room table in the company of others. We sit too much and move too little.

It turns out that health springs largely from old-fashioned behaviors—eating wholesome food, enjoying friends, relaxing, getting enough sleep, moving our bodies, and using natural remedies to heal.

The goal of this book is to help you get back to the basic lifestyle measures that point you toward a healthy, vibrant future.

We provide lots of practical information on preventing and managing ailments. You'll find time-tested recipes and lifestyle tips—all designed to give you sometimes quick, always natural, ways to soothe, calm, and heal.

We hope you enjoy this book. May it enlighten you, guiding you along natural and simple paths to your healthy future.

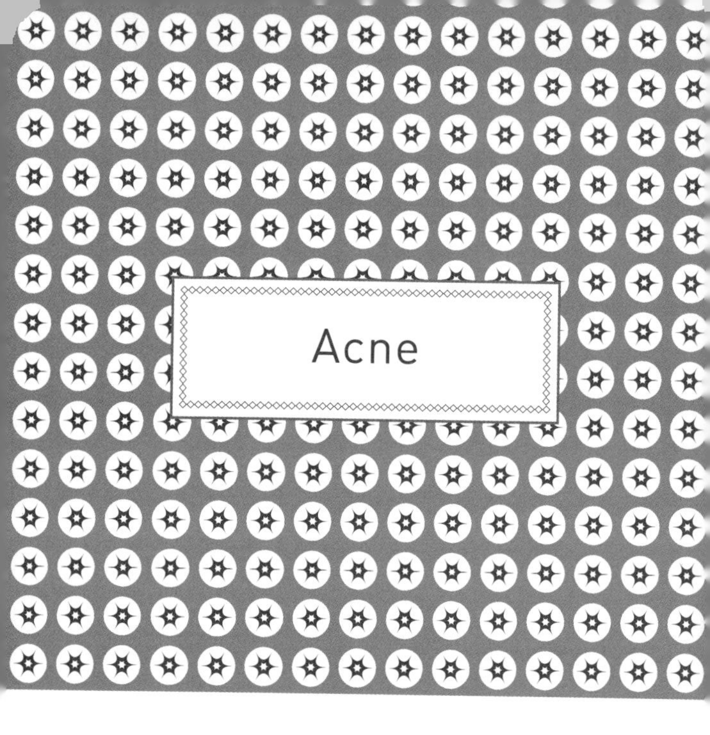

“Out damn'd spot”—Lady Macbeth's anguished cry in Shakespeare's *Macbeth*—might also be the mantra of acne sufferers. For all the effort spent hunting for medications and remedies and all the dismay caused by skin eruptions and breakouts, acne ranks right up there with the most troubling common ailments.

Acne is, for many teens, a rite of passage. About the time girls and boys enter puberty, acne may strike. Acne (*acne vulgaris*) goes by many names: zits, blackheads, pimples, bumps, blemishes, and more. Adolescence marks a time of hormonal surges, including an abundance of male hormones from the adrenal gland. Among other actions, these hormones increase the skin's oil production. If the pores to the oils glands become clogged, localized inflammation and infection—redness, swelling, and pus—can result. In severe cases, doctors sometimes prescribe oral antibiotics or synthetic vitamin A derivatives (Accutane, taken internally, and Retin-A, applied externally).

Part of the trouble in treating acne is that it can strike not only in the teen years but in adulthood as well.

Essential Oil Lotion

"I've had my kids apply these essential oils directly to acne. Aloe adds a soothing element." ~LBW

2 drops pure tea tree or lavender essential oil
1 teaspoon (5 g) Aloe vera gel

PREPARATION AND USE:

Blend the tea tree essential oil with the aloe gel. Dot the mixture on blemishes using a cotton swab or clean finger.

YIELD: 1 APPLICATION

How it works: Tea tree and lavender are both anti-inflammatory and antimicrobial. Lavender smells nicer and can be applied without dilution. Aloe vera is also anti-inflammatory and antimicrobial. In addition, it reduces discomfort and speeds healing. Topical applications of 5 per- cent tea tree oil gel have been proven as effective as benzoyl peroxide (Oxy-5) and other commer- cially available products.

Apple Cider Vinegar Wash

Some people apply vinegar undiluted, but we recommend cutting it with water. You can always build back up to full strength.

½ cup (120 ml) water

2 tablespoons (28 ml) apple cider vinegar

PREPARATION AND USE:

Pour the water and vinegar into a small, clean bowl. Stir to combine. With a cotton swab or cotton ball, dab the diluted vinegar on each blemish. (Use one swab or ball per blemish to keep infection from spreading.) The application may briefly sting, but that should soon stop. Apply nightly for best results.

YIELD: 1 APPLICATION

How it works: Vinegar contains acetic acid, which is an antiseptic and helps regulate skin acidity.

Warning: Because undiluted vinegar may irritate the skin, always start with a 1:8 dilution of vinegar to water (e.g., 2 tablespoons [28 ml] of vinegar to 1 cup [235 ml] of water) and build up to 1:4 and, if possible, to vinegar only.

Yogurt Honey Mask

¼ cup (60 g) plain yogurt

1 tablespoon (20 g) honey

2 strawberries

PREPARATION AND USE:

In a small bowl, blend the yogurt and honey. Mash the strawberries and fold into the yogurt mixture. Pull back your hair and wash your face with warm water. Use a cotton ball to spread the mask onto your face. Recline for 10 minutes while the fruit and milk acids do their work. Wash with cool water and pat dry with a clean towel.

YIELD: 1 application

How it works: Yogurt contains lactic acid and strawberries contain several fruit acids, primarily citric acid. These acids help remove dead skin cells and unclog pores. Honey is antibacterial, anti-inflammatory, and antioxidant.

Note: Alternatively, dab on straight honey, allow it to dry, and then rinse.

Pineapple Refresh

1 fresh pineapple

PREPARATION AND USE:

Slice away the sides of the pineapple, separating the fruit from the rind. Set the fruit aside in a bowl. Rub the inside of the rind on your face. Mash a single slice of pineapple and rub it onto your face. Let the pineapple juices work for about 15 minutes—while you enjoy eating the fruit. Wash your face and pat it dry with a clean towel. Repeat weekly as needed.

YIELD: 1 application

How it works: Pineapple contains an anti-inflammatory enzyme called bromelain and fruit acids (mainly citric acid), which gently exfoliate the skin, unblock pores, and dry excess skin oil.

(A number of over-the-counter anti-acne products contain a type of fruit acid called alpha-hydroxy acid.) One study found that a commercially prepared fruit acid product, applied to the face every two weeks for six months, decreased the number of pimples.

Warning: Do not apply pineapple to your skin if you're allergic to it. If you develop any redness or irritation, stop.

Bitter Greens Salad

Be creative with this natural cleanser by trying greens you've never used before.

½ cup (28 g) fresh dandelion greens
½ cup (10 g) arugula
½ cup (20 g) radicchio
½ cup (25 g) endive
½ cup (150 g) fresh or canned artichoke hearts

PREPARATION AND USE:

Tear the greens into bite-size pieces. Slice the artichoke hearts. Mix all the ingredients together in a salad. Add other favorite vegetables but avoid adding ingredients with sugars, which may cause skin flare-ups.

YIELD: 2 servings

How it works: Bitter foods stimulate the liver, the organ that breaks down hormones and many other chemicals so they can more easily be cleared from the body.

Herbal Steam Bag

This herbal remedy can also be used as a soothing facial anytime you need it.

1 quart (946 ml) water
1 tablespoon (2 g) crushed dried calendula (also called pot marigold) flowers
1 tablespoon (2 g) dried elderflowers
3 drops lavender essential oil

PREPARATION AND USE:

Bring water to a boil in a kettle. Put the calendula flowers and elderflowers in a large, heatproof bowl and add the water, covering the flowers. Add the lavender oil and stir to combine. Lower your head over the bowl and cover it completely with a towel. Allow the steam to work for 15 minutes or until it abates. Rinse your face with cool water.

YIELD: 1 application

How it works: Calendula and elderflower have anti-inflammatory and antiseptic properties.

Note: You'll find dried herbal flowers in bulk at most health food stores. Also, although calendula (*Calendula officinalis*) also goes by the common name of pot marigold, it is not the same as marigold (*Tagetes erecta, T. patula*, and other species).

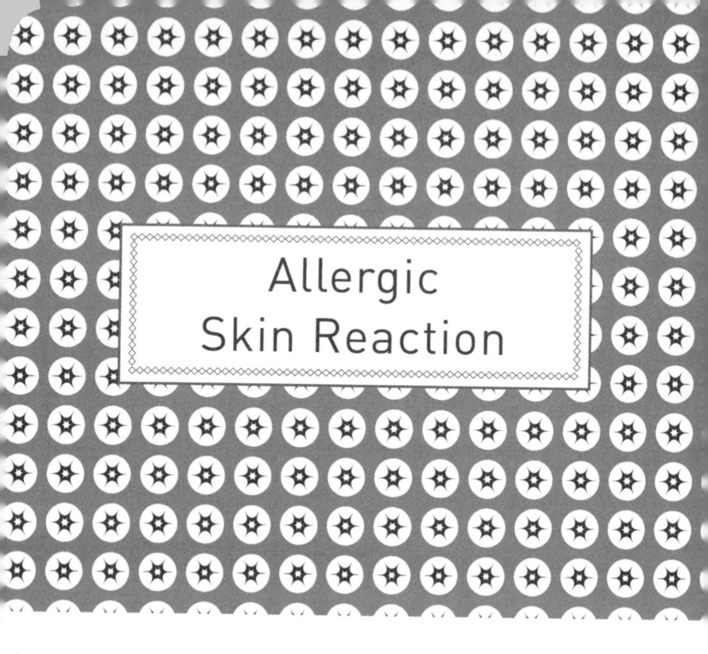

Allergic Skin Reaction

The skin is the body's largest organ. A number of things can trigger local skin inflammation, or dermatitis, in sensitive people. In contact dermatitis, the offending agents come into direct contact with the skin. Examples include poison ivy, nickel jewelry, sheep's lanolin, topical antibiotics, and ingredients in detergents and body-care products. Radiation administered to cancer patients can also cause dermatitis.

Some people have eczema, also called atopic dermatitis, a condition that tends to run in families, along with hay fever and asthma. Affected patches of skin are red, itchy, scaly, and thickened, and in some cases oozing and crusty. Allergens that provoke the inflammation may be difficult or impossible to identify.

Hives is another skin condition often caused by an allergic reaction. Red, raised itchy patches of skin appear suddenly and may disappear as quickly as they came. Caused by a release of histamine in response to an allergen, hives can be triggered by just about anything—food, sun, dust mites, stress, medication, and more.

Treatment for any of these conditions depends upon the underlying cause. If your watch's nickel backing left a red, crusty patch on your wrist, you'll need to replace it. If you're allergic to the antibiotic you're taking, you may need to switch medications and remember to never take that antibiotic again (as the reaction could be more severe next time around). If you're allergic to bee venom and are stung, you'll need an epinephrine injection. If you are prone to hives, a simple antihistamine can often calm the allergic reaction. If you have eczema, your doctor will probably advise switching to hypoallergenic personal care products and laundry detergent, keeping your skin hydrated, and prescription anti-inflammatory creams for flare-ups.

RECIPES TO TREAT ALLERGIC SKIN REACTIONS

Salad Dressing to Foil Inflammation

1 part olive oil

1 part flaxseed oil

1 part balsamic vinegar

1 part apple cider vinegar

PREPARATION AND USE:

Combine all the ingredients in a dressing shaker and shake vigorously ten times. Pour over salad and toss.

YIELD: 4 to 6 servings

How it works: You may think that eating oil will cause your skin to break out; in fact, oil is an anti-inflammatory. The omega-3 fatty acids in fish oil are especially effective in retarding inflammatory reactions in cells.

LIFESTYLE TIP

For an extra jolt of good-for-you oils, never consume cod liver oil. It contains too much vitamin A for your system and can even cause a bleeding disorder. Instead, opt for other sources of healthy oils. Add walnuts and avocados to salad. Add hemp seeds to cereal and smoothies. Eat oily fish (salmon, mackerel, sardines, etc.) at least once a week. Or take a daily EPA/DHA capsule.

Colloidal Oatmeal Bath

2 to 3 cups (160 to 240 g) regular or colloidal oats

PREPARATION AND USE:

If using regular oats, pour them into a food processor, coffee grinder, or blender and blend to a powder. This turns them into colloidal oats.

Pour the oats into warm, running bathwater. Disperse oats with your hand. (Alternatively, pour the oats into a sock, bag, or bandana to contain the particles and help with cleanup and place the sock in the bathwater.) Climb in and soak for at least 15 minutes. (Avoid using soap, which only dries and further irritates the skin.) After leaving the bath, pat your skin dry with a clean towel.

YIELD: 1 application

How it works: Oats have antioxidant and anti-inflammatory activity. Applied topically, oats moisturize the skin and decrease itching. The gooeyness you feel when you squeeze the sock is caused by the complex carbohydrates in the oats.

Note: You can make a large batch of colloidal oats and store in a tightly sealed jar or tin in a cool, dry place.

Afterbath Natural Moisturizer

¼ cup (55 ml) Aloe vera gel
¼ cup (60 ml) high-quality oil (olive, almond, coconut, apricot, or grapeseed)
12 drops German chamomile essential oil

PREPARATION AND USE:

In a clean bowl, whisk together the aloe gel and oil. Blend in the German chamomile oil. Immediately after bathing or showering, while your skin is still damp, apply a generous amount to your skin with clean fingers. Allow a couple of minutes for the moisturizer to absorb before getting dressed.

YIELD: Multiple applications

How it works:

- Aloe vera gel is anti-inflammatory, soothing, and hydrating. Lab studies indicate that aloe can promote healing and may reduce inflammation in eczema.
- German chamomile (*Matricaria recutita*) has chemicals that reduce inflammation and allergies. More specifically, the flavonoids quercetin and apigenin inhibit the release of histamine from immune cells called mast cells. Lab studies indicate that it improves eczema-like skin conditions. Essential oil of chamomile looks blue, due to a potent anti-inflammatory chemical called chamazulene.

Note: Store leftover moisturizer in a clean, dry jar and throw it away after two weeks when it's time for a fresh recipe.

Soothing Oat Paste

1 tablespoon (5 g) colloidal oatmeal

1 teaspoon (5 g) baking soda

Drops of water, as needed

PREPARATION AND USE:

In a small bowl, stir together the colloidal oatmeal and baking soda until blended. Gradually add just enough water to form a paste. Apply to irritated areas with clean fingers. Once dry, rinse it off with warm water.

YIELD: 1 application

How it works: The antioxidant and anti-inflammatory activities in oatmeal relieve itching. Baking soda neutralizes the acids that promote itchy skin.

Fact or Myth?

STRESS CAN AGGRAVATE ECZEMA.

Yes! To help counteract a breakout and increasing irritation, take a long walk, bike, or swim; do the Stress Less exercise (see page 119) in a quiet room; or meditate.

Jewelweed Rub

Jewelweed (Impatiens capensis) *is a tall, stemmed plant with orange and yellow trumpet-shaped flowers, usually found growing wild near streams and in deep shade in the woods. My family keeps a batch of this handy during poison ivy season. (Jewelweed can sometimes be found at nurseries, but don't confuse it with the shade-tolerant garden annual Impatiens walleriana, also known as "Busy Lizzy." That one will not help your poison ivy.) ~ BHS*

1 quart (946 ml) water (or more if you have lots of jewelweed)
Armful of jewelweed

PREPARATION AND USE:

Bring the water to a boil in a big pot. Turn off the heat. Put the jewelweed in the pot, cover it, and let it steep for at least 30 minutes. Pour the mixture (a deep brown tea) into a gallon jar or into icecube trays and freeze. Rub on the poison ivy rash as soon as you experience the first signs of itching.

YIELD: Enough for dozens of applications

How it works: Urushiol, an oily resin in the sap of poison ivy, poison oak, and poison sumac, causes an allergic reaction in those who are sensitive to it. Jewelweed has strong anti-inflammatory properties. It acts on urushiol to relieve the itching and blisters and halt the spread of the rash.

Sage Skin Wash

1 cup (235 ml) water

1 tablespoon (2 g) dried sage

PREPARATION AND USE:

In a small pot, bring the water to a boil and then pour into a cup. Add the dried sage, cover, and let steep for at least 15 minutes. Strain and allow to cool to room temperature. Apply to the affected area with a clean cloth. Allow the skin to dry before getting dressed. Do not rinse off the sage mixture.

YIELD: 1 application

How it works: In a 2011 study in Japan, researchers used sage and rosemary, among other herbal extracts, on dermatitis lesions on mice and found that repeated applications significantly healed the skin lesions.

STRESS CAN AGGRAVATE ECZEMA.

- You develop a rash around your eyes, mouth, genitals, or over much of your body from poison ivy or poison oak.
- Skin inflammation worsens or becomes infected, as evidenced by increased redness, heat, and pus.
- Fever or other signs of more serious illness accompany skin inflammation.

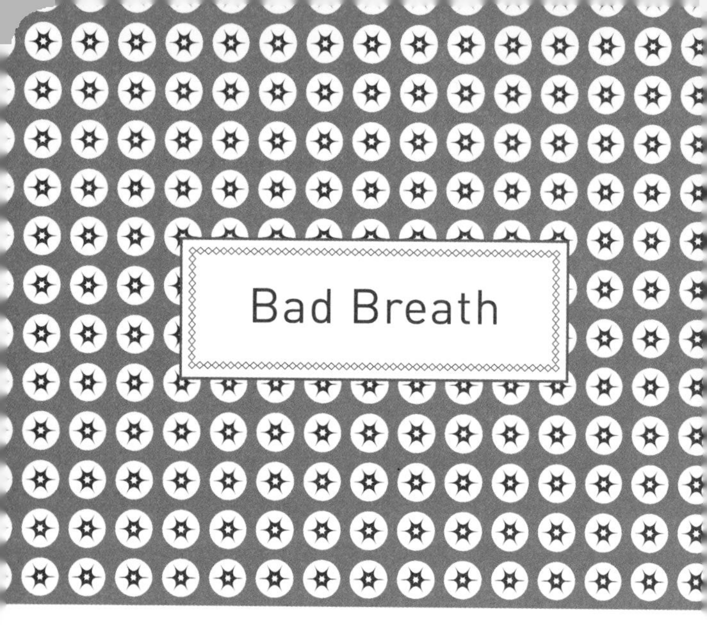

Bad breath affects an estimated 25 to 30 percent of the world's population. About 2.4 percent of adults have chronic halitosis. The majority of the time, the origin is in the mouth. Examples include gum disease, dental cavities, coated tongue (sometimes a white or yellow layer blankets the tongue, usually due to inflammation), and poor oral hygiene. Beneficial microorganisms normally line our entire intestinal tract, peacefully coexisting with us. However, oral diseases involve proliferation of certain microorganisms that produce sulfurous smells.

Smokers have bad breath. Food and drink, such as onions, garlic, coffee, and alcohol, can temporarily taint breath. Other peoples' reactions are tempered by whether they have also indulged in the same food or drink and whether they happen to dislike that smell. Some say vegetarians have sweeter breath than meat eaters. That difference has to do with how mouth microbes act on amino acids (the building blocks in protein) and digestive processes deeper in the intestinal tract.

Because saliva has an antimicrobial effect, having a dry mouth sours breath. Advanced age, stress, depression, mouth breathing, alcohol abuse, certain medications, diabetes, and Sjögren syndrome (an autoimmune disease wherein white blood cells attack glands that make saliva and tears) diminish saliva. Reduced nighttime saliva production also causes morning breath.

In addition, malnutrition contributes to overall ill health and bad breath. Insufficient consumption of carbohydrates or severe caloric restriction leaves your body no choice but to break down fat, which gives your breath a telltale fruity odor. Uncontrolled diabetes also creates disturbances in oral health.

Such infections as sore throat and sinusitis cause halitosis. So do stomach and intestinal disorders, such as heartburn, stomach inflammation and ulcers, and lactose intolerance. Treatment involves correcting the underlying disorder.

Citrus Fresh Breath

The rind tastes bitter at first bite, but chewing it gives your mouth a natural, refreshing zing.

1 organic lemon or orange

PREPARATION AND USE:

Wash the rind thoroughly and tear off a piece. Chew for a flavorful, mouth-freshening burst.

YIELD: 1 application

How it works: Citric acid will stimulate the salivary glands to create saliva, which is a natural breath freshener.

Minty Mouth-Freshening Tea

2 tablespoons (12 g) loose green tea, or

2 tea bags

1 teaspoon (2 g) crushed fresh mint leaves

1 cinnamon stick

2 cups (475 ml) boiled water

PREPARATION AND USE:

Add the tea, mint leaves, and cinnamon to the boiled water. Steep for 5 minutes. Remove the tea bags, if using, and strain out the herbs. Sip and enjoy!

YIELD: 1 large or 2 small servings

How it works: Green tea has antibacterial compounds. Cinnamon is antimicrobial and aromatic. The oils in mint fight mouth bacteria that cause halitosis.

Crunch It

1 cup (150 g) apple chunks

1 cup (110 g) grated carrot

1 cup (120 g) diced celery

½ cup (60 g) dried cranberries

½ cup (60 g) crushed walnuts

3 to 5 tablespoons (45 to 75 g) plain nonfat yogurt

Ground cinnamon

PREPARATION AND USE:

Mix the apple, carrot, celery, cranberries, and walnuts together in a large bowl. Add the yogurt by the tablespoon (15 g) to moisten the mixture and hold it together slightly. Divide between two plates, sprinkle with cinnamon, and serve.

YIELD: 2 servings

How it works: Raw, crunchy foods clean the teeth. Apples contain pectin, which helps control food odors. It also promotes saliva, which cleanses breath. Cinnamon is antimicrobial. Yogurt contains the type of bacteria you want in your intestinal tract. Studies show that the active bacteria and cultures in yogurt help reduce odor-causing bacteria in the mouth.

Peroxide Swish

Hydrogen peroxide is a versatile cleansing agent, in the right doses. Be sure to cut it with water before using.

2 tablespoons (30 ml) hydrogen peroxide

2 tablespoons (30 ml) water

PREPARATION AND USE:

Mix the hydrogen peroxide and water in a clean glass. Swish in your mouth for 30 seconds and then spit out. Rinse twice a day, once in the morning and once in the evening.

How it works: Hydrogen peroxide's oxygen content kills the bacteria in your mouth that cause bad breath.

LIFESTYLE TIP

When nothing else is available, swish fresh, cool water around in your mouth. Water freshens breath and makes you feel better in general.

Mouthwash in a Minute

We love the fresh and natural taste of this mouthwash—and it's alcohol-free, unlike so many off-the-shelf products. Do not swallow it!

1 cup (235 ml) water

1 teaspoon (5 g) baking soda

3 drops peppermint essential oil

PREPARATION AND USE:

Mix together all the ingredients. Pour into a clean glass jar with a tight-fitting lid, cap, and shake. Use a small amount to rinse your mouth for about 30 seconds. Spit out—do not swallow.

YIELD: Several rinses; make a fresh batch after a few days, or alter the recipe to make a little at a time.

How it works: Peppermint is antimicrobial. Baking soda changes the pH (acid) levels in the mouth, creating an antiodor environment.

Yogurt Breath Blaster

1 cup (230 g) vanilla yogurt

1 cup (170 g) sliced strawberries

¼ cup (30 g) chopped walnuts

Sprigs of mint

PREPARATION AND USE:

Combine the yogurt, strawberries, and walnuts in a small bowl. Top with mint sprigs and serve.

YIELD: 1 serving

How it works: Studies say that yogurt's active bacteria may help control the mouth bacteria that release malodorous chemicals, such as hydrogen sulfide. In one study, researchers found that eating 6 ounces (170 g) of yogurt a day reduced levels of this gas.

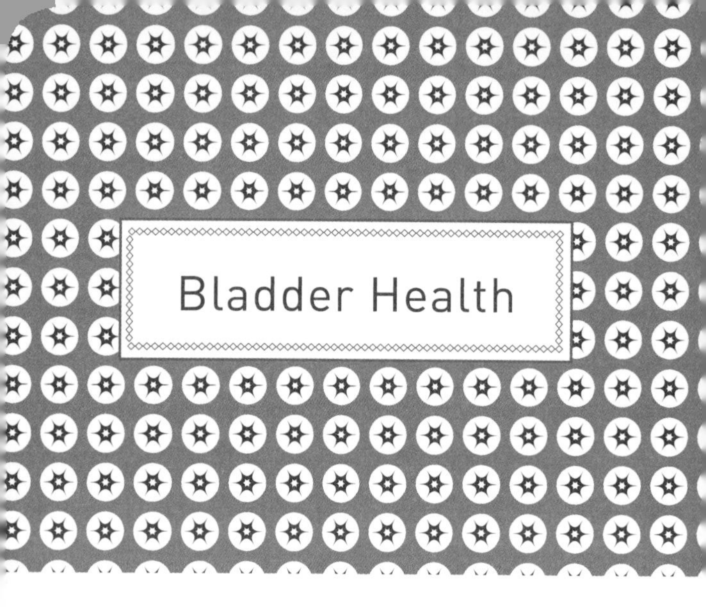

Bladder Health

If you're a woman, chances are fifty-fifty that you've had at least one episode of cystitis, better known as a bladder infection. Urinary tract infections, or UTIs (infection anywhere along the urinary system from the kidney to the urethra), are the most common bacterial infections in women. Within the category of UTIs, bladder infections top the list—so much so that people use UTI and bladder infection interchangeably.

The reason such infections are predominantly a female affliction has to do with relative shortness of the urethra (the tube that transports fluids from the kidneys to the genitals for removal). Bowel bacteria such as E. coli, the usual cause of UTIs, simply don't need to travel far to reach the bladder. And bacteria are, the most common cause of acute bladder infections.

Classic symptoms include burning with urination, increased frequency of urination, an urgent need to urinate (even if the bladder isn't very full), nighttime urination, and discomfort above the pubic bone. The urine may be cloudy and foul smelling. Previously toilet-trained children may have "accidents." Young children may have only nonspecific symptoms, such as a mild fever, irritability, poor feeding, and restless sleep.

At the doctor's office, you'll be asked to provide a clean midstream urine sample. Because small children can't usually provide an uncontaminated urine sample, doctors typically insert a catheter into their bladder or a needle through the skin of the lower abdomen into the bladder. A urine sample is taken and then analyzed. If bacteria are present, oral antibiotics are prescribed.

Antibiotics not only quickly stamp out the infection but prevent the bacteria from ascending to the kidneys. Kidney infection (pyelonephritis) is serious. Symptoms include flank pain, fever, and chills. It can scar the kidneys, leading to problems such as high blood pressure and kidney failure. Treatment often requires hospitalization, with intravenous fluids and antibiotics.

After a bladder infection, your doctor will probably ask you to return for a repeat urine culture to make sure no bacteria survived. Boys younger than twelve months of age with a first-time infection and little girls with more than one infection usually undergo tests to check for anatomical abnormalities that would lead to repeated infection and kidney damage.

RECIPES FOR BLADDER HEALTH

Before recommending recipes for bladder health, we'd like to stress the importance of proper medical treatment of UTIs. These remedies are not intended as a replacement for antibiotic treatment. They may, however, help prevent recurrent infections.

Cranberry Mocktail

1 cup (235 ml) unsweetened cranberry juice

¾ cup (175 ml) carbonated (sparkling) water

2 lemon slices

2 teaspoons (14 g) honey

PREPARATION AND USE:

Mix together all the ingredients. Aim to drink both servings of this cocktail in one day.

YIELD: 2 servings

Recipe Variation: Substitute apple juice or sparkling cider for the carbonated water and omit the honey.

How it works: Research studies show that cranberry juice and concentrated cranberry tablets reduce UTI recurrences. Also, the tannins that create the characteristic mouth-puckering effect of cranberries are also astringent in the urinary system. (Astringents tighten tissues and are thought to reduce surface irritation and inflammation. Cranberry is acidic, but it takes a lot of volume to acidify the urine enough to kill bacteria.)

Note: The daily volume of cranberry juice used in studies ranges from 2 tablespoons (30 ml) to 1 cup (235 ml) of pure cranberry juice. Higher doses can loosen stools. If you find you can't stomach cranberry juice, try taking concentrated cranberry in capsule form as directed on the label. Be aware that commercially prepared cranberry juice drinks contain added water and sugar.

Do not combine cranberry with the blood-thinning medication warfarin (Coumadin) without first discussing with your doctor. Case reports suggest cranberry may augment the effect of Coumadin, further reducing the ability of blood to clot. However, the problem has not been detected in clinical trials.

LIFESTYLE TIP

Use warmth. Fill a hot water bottle or turn on a heating pad and place it over your lower abdomen. Heat improves blood flow, relaxes muscles, and helps relieve dis- comfort from a bladder infection.

Beneficial Blueberry Smoothie

1 cup (230 g) plain yogurt

½ cup (75 g) blueberries

½ cup (120 ml) "crabapple" juice
(cranberry juice and apple juice combined)

PREPARATION AND USE:

Mix all the ingredients in a blender. Enjoy.

YIELD: 1 serving

How it works: Blueberries belong to the same plant family as cranberries. They, too, contain flavonoids that inhibit the adhesion of bacteria to bodily surfaces. The yogurt contains beneficial bacteria (probiotics) that can help restore normal bowel bacteria if you've taken antibiotics to treat a UTI. However, the research is inconclusive as to whether probiotics (taken by mouth or used intravaginally) help prevent recurrent cystitis.

Nutrient-Rich Dandelion Tea

If in season, pick spring dandelion leaves—as long as they're not exposed to pesticides or growing near a road. Bundle and hang to dry in a warm, dim place. Once dry to the touch, crumble the leaves; place in a clean, dry jar; and store in the cupboard. You may also be able to find them dried or fresh at a natural food store.

1 quart (946 ml) water

3 tablespoons (4.5 g) dried, chopped dandelion leaves

1 teaspoon (0.5 g) chopped dried peppermint leaves, or 2 teaspoons (4 g) fresh, chopped

Honey, as needed

PREPARATION AND USE:

Bring the water to a boil in a saucepan. Turn off the heat and add the dandelion and peppermint. Cover and steep for 20 minutes. Strain. Sweeten with honey to taste. Drink throughout the day.

YIELD: 4 servings

How it works: Dandelion is nutrient-rich and gently increases urine output. You can also enjoy the tender greens in salads, steamed, or sautéed. Peppermint is antispasmodic and also tastes pleasant.

Yogurt-Berry Ice

This delicious dessert is smooth and creamy and delivers friendly bacteria to your system. For a drinkable smoothie version, see the variation below.

2 cups (about 200 g) frozen mixed berries, or ⅔ bag (16-ounces, or 455 g)

½ cup (115 g) plain yogurt

3 tablespoons (60 g) honey

⅛ teaspoon almond extract

PREPARATION AND USE:

Allow the berries to thaw for 7 to 10 minutes. Pour into a blender or processor and grind until the fruit pieces look like shaved ice. While the blender is running, add the yogurt, honey, and almond extract. Continue blending until the mixture is creamy. Eat immediately, as the texture will change when refrozen.

YIELD: 4 servings

Recipe Variation: For drinkable smoothies, add ½ cup (120 ml) of almond milk.

How it works: Antibiotics effectively treat UTIs. However, they also kill some of the normal, friendly bacteria in the bowel. Probiotics, taken in supplement form, help recolonize normal bacteria and prevent side effects such as diarrhea. Yogurt and other fermented foods, which contain beneficial bacteria, may also help.

Soothing Sitz Bath

If using oats for this recipe, be sure to put them in a coffee mill and grind them to a powder; otherwise, they'll clog the drain.

2 to 3 cups (576 to 864 g) salt(442 to 663 g), baking soda, or (160 to 240 g) colloidal oatmeal

PREPARATION AND USE:

Fill your bathtub with water as warm as you can stand it. Pour in the salt, baking soda, or oatmeal and disperse. Soak for at least 30 minutes.

YIELD: 1 application

Recipe Variation: You can also use 2 to 3 cups (475 to 700 ml) of vinegar, but don't combine it with baking soda, or you'll have a fizzy reaction.

How it works: The warmth of the water with the soothing ingredients helps relax the urethra. Baking soda and salt can soothe irritated membranes. Oatmeal has anti-inflammatory properties and promotes wound healing. Vinegar, which you can also add, is mildly acidic and helps relieve irritation of the vagina and urethra.

Note: Clean your feet before sitting in the tub so you do not introduce new bacteria.

Encourage children who have trouble urinating because of pain to go ahead and squat in the water and let it go. Then have them step out of the tub immediately.

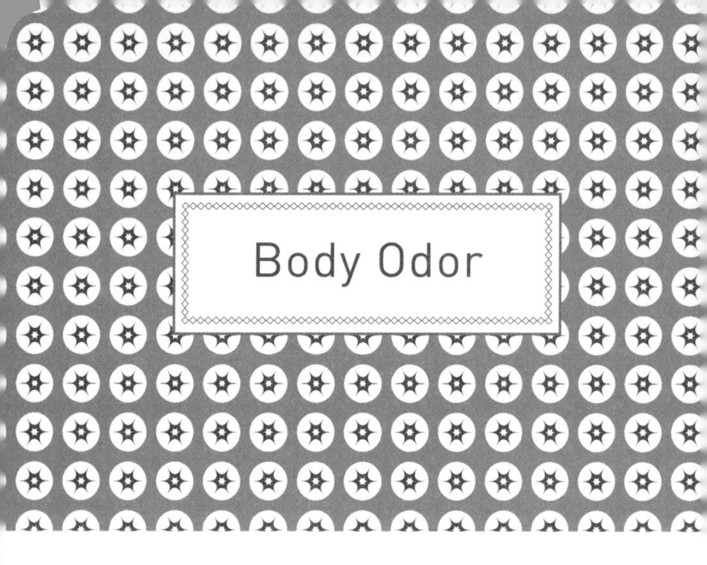

Aromatic appeal is, to some extent, subjective. The sense of smell is primal, mysterious, and deeply personal. Compared to that of most other mammals, our olfactory perception is dull. Yet, it remains important for survival. It helps us detect smoke, identify whether food has gone bad, and determine whether we or our clothes need washing.

Odor receptors in the nose connect swiftly to deep and ancient parts of the brain, including those involved in strong emotions and memory formation and retrieval. Mothers and babies of all mammalian species recognize one another by scent. Scent figures in our choice of a mate. In fact, body odors provide subconscious information about a potential mate's genetic compatibility, social status, and reproductive vigor. Fluctuations in female hormones temper a woman's olfactory sensitivity.

What creates a person's signature aroma? A lot of things: diet, overall state of health, age, emotional state, levels of certain hormones, hygiene, and some medications. Some diseases create characteristic chemicals detectable on skin and in breath. Examples of illnesses that alter skin smells include infectious diseases (for example, tuberculosis and scarlet fever), scurvy (vitamin C deficiency), and schizophrenia.

Americans tend to be particularly preoccupied with body odor. The armpits are the usual source. Armpit sweat, which is richer in proteins and fats than secretions from the sweat glands covering most of your skin, doesn't stink until bacteria that normally colonize your skin break down chemicals in sweat into acids. What can you do?

- Bathe regularly, paying special attention to your armpits and bottom. You don't need to use harsh antibacterial soaps. In fact, some of the antibacterial chemicals (e.g., triclosan) aren't good for you or the environment. Use a mild soap with a natural (plant-derived) fragrance.

- Wear natural fabrics. These allow your sweat to evaporate freely. It's when your armpits are hot, sweaty, and lacking in oxygen that odor-causing bacteria thrive. In winter, you can't beat wool for warm and wicking action.

- Eat more fruits and vegetables. Vegetarians are said to smell sweeter than people who eat a lot of meat.

- Harness the antibacterial and aromatic properties of plant essential oils. See the recipes throughout this chapter.

Take a Powder

Using just two pantry ingredients, this recipe is quick, easy, and effective. Essential oils add sweetness to this natural remedy.

¼ cup (55 g) baking soda

¼ cup (32 g) cornstarch

PREPARATION AND USE:

Mix the baking soda and cornstarch together in a small glass dish. Apply to underarms with a clean makeup pad. Apply to feet and the insides of shoes to sop up foot odors.

YIELD: Multiple applications

Recipe Variation: Add 10 to 12 drops of lavender or another favorite essential oil per ½ cup (87 g) of the mixture. Drop the oil into a bowl, pour the powder mixture into a sieve, and shake it into the oil, gradually mixing the two to blend.

How it works: Baking soda is a natural odor eliminator. Cornstarch absorbs excess moisture.

Warning: Be careful not to inhale the particles.

Coconut Tea Tree Deodorizer

This recipe, used with permission from Rachel Hoff of Dog Island Farm, an urban farm northeast of San Francisco, is easy to make and safe for you and the environment.

2 tablespoons (28 g) virgin coconut oil

1 tablespoon (14 g) grated beeswax

8 drops tea tree essential oil

2 tablespoons (28 g) baking soda

2 tablespoons (16 g) cornstarch

PREPARATION AND USE:

In a saucepan over low heat, melt the coconut oil and beeswax. (Alternatively, you can use the double-boiler method to make sure you don't burn the oil.) Once melted, remove from the heat. Immediately add the essential oil, baking soda, and cornstarch and stir to combine. (If you wait, the cooling beeswax will harden the oil, making it difficult to mix in the dry ingredients.) Pour the mixture into a clean, dry, empty push-style deodorant container (recycle a used one). Use a spatula or butter knife to pack in the mixture and smooth over the top.

YIELD: Enough for 1 medium-size deodorant container

How it works: Virgin coconut oil is antibacterial and an emollient. Tea tree oil is antimicrobial. Beeswax holds the mixture together, smells pleasant, and soothes irritated skin.

Note: Alternatively, buy beeswax pastilles (pellet-size pieces of beeswax). If you bought a 1-ounce (28 g) piece of beeswax, simply cut it in half. Save the other half for later.

Lavender-Apple Cider Vinegar Wash

A refreshing spray of this underarm elixir has postshower power.

¼ cup (60 ml) apple cider vinegar

6 drops lavender essential oil

PREPARATION AND USE:

Place the ingredients in a small, clean spray bottle, cap, and shake. Spritz on underarms after a shower or bath.

YIELD: Multiple applications

How it works: Apple cider vinegar lowers the pH level of the skin (that is, makes the skin more acidic), discouraging bacteria that turn body sweat into body odor. Lavender discourages bacterial growth and adds a scent-ual lift.

Sage Therapy

This freshening agent can be grown year-round in your backyard. Be sure to chop or crush the sage—you want the plants in small pieces to increase their surface area of exposure to the solvent, in this case vinegar.

2 tablespoons (5 g) crushed or chopped fresh sage

¼ cup (60 ml) apple cider vinegar

PREPARATION AND USE:

Combine the sage and vinegar in the small, clean jar. Cap and shake the mixture until the sage is thoroughly soaked. Place the mixture in the pantry or cabinet for about a week. (This allows the vinegar to extract the essence of the sage.) When the vinegar smells strongly of sage, the potion is ready. Strain the mixture through cheesecloth and pour it into a small, clean spray bottle. Spritz your underarms, feet, or other body parts prone to odor.

YIELD: Multiple applications

How it works: Sage has a drying effect and is antimicrobial. Combined with the pH-reducing apple cider vinegar, it makes a perfect elixir for reducing perspiration and body odor.

Essentially Yours

Essential oils not only fight bacteria and microbes, keeping you at your freshest, but they infuse your home with soothing scent.

¼ cup (60 ml) witch hazel

1 tablespoon (15 ml) vodka

10 drops tea tree oil

10 drops lavender essential oil

5 drops eucalyptus essential oil

5 drops sage essential oil

PREPARATION AND USE:

In a clean spray bottle, mix the witch hazel and vodka. Add all the essential oils. Cap and shake the bottle until the ingredients are completely blended. Spritz away at those odiferous body parts.

YIELD: Multiple applications

How it works: Witch hazel is astringent and antiseptic; vodka is antibacterial. Lavender, eucalyptus, and sage essential oils are antibacterial, while tea tree oil is antimicrobial. Sage also has drying properties.

Refreshing Bath Fizzie

This recipe comes from one of the staff at a Denver herb store called Apothecary Tinctura. It leaves you smelling clean and feeling refreshed.

¼ to ½ cup (60 to 120 ml) witch hazel

½ cup (115 g) citric acid

1 cup (220 g) baking soda

15 drops eucalyptus essential oil

10 drops bay laurel essential oil

PREPARATION AND USE:

Pour the witch hazel into a small, clean spray bottle. In a small bowl, combine the citric acid and baking soda. Add the essential oils to the powder one drop at a time, stirring constantly to distribute evenly. Pick up the mixture in your hands and spritz two times with witch hazel. Keep shaping and spritzing the material with your hands until you have a ball that's moist but not soggy. Press into muffin tins, filling halfway. Once dry, pop out the fizzies and store in a tightly capped jar. Add one fizzie to a warm bath.

YIELD: 6 refreshing bath fizzies

How it works: The citric acid and baking soda are delivery systems for the refreshing aromatic essential oils. Eucalyptus and bay laurel essential oils are antibacterial agents that help counter odor-causing skin bacteria.

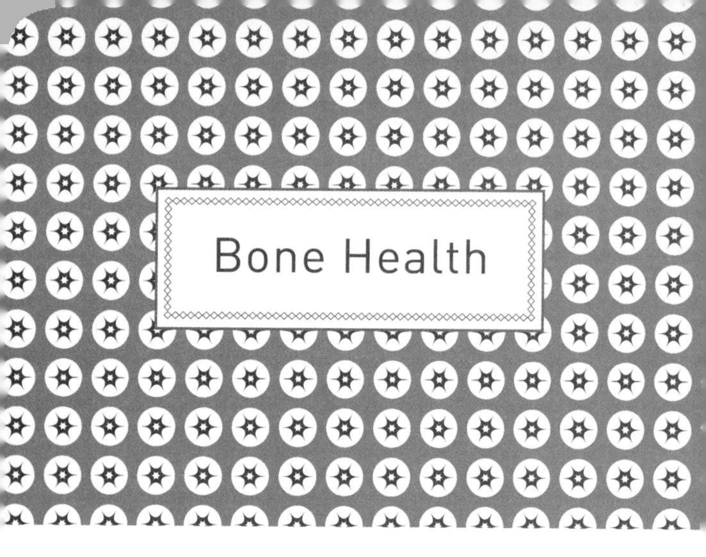

Bone Health

Our bones define us, make us beautiful (think Audrey Hepburn or Jessica Chastain), provide the leverage for movement, and allow us to stand upright. We build bone until our third decade. After that, our bone loss outpaces bone deposition.

For women, bone loss accelerates at menopause. In comparison, men tend to have denser bones to start with and their loss is less marked. But even though osteoporosis, a condition in which bones become more porous and fragile, is more common in older women, men are far from immune. In adults age fifty and older, 16 percent of women and 4 percent of men have osteoporosis. More than 40 million Americans either have osteoporosis or borderline low bone mass.

The result can be painful and debilitating bone fractures. Hip fractures can lead to disability, loss of independence, and premature death. Early identification with bone density tests and prompt treatment with lifestyle changes, supplements, and medications can avert such disasters. Testing is particularly important because osteoporosis is silent, causing few symptoms until a bone shatters.

A number of risk factors increase your risk of osteoporosis. Some you can't control, such as being female, postmenopausal, having a small frame, being white or Asian, having a family history of osteoporosis, being chronically ill or bedridden, and taking certain medications. Medications include certain antiseizure and anticancer medications, antidepressants (specifically selective serotonin reuptake inhibitors), aluminum-containing antacids, proton pump inhibitors (stomach-acid-reducing drugs, such as Prilosec), and corticosteroids (cortisone and derivatives).

Artichoke Heart Salad

¼ red onion, sliced thinly

2 tablespoons (30 ml) fresh lemon juice

1 pound (455 g) asparagus

1 tablespoon (15 ml) olive oil

1 jar (13 ounces, or 365 g) artichoke hearts, sliced in half

½ pint (225 g) cherry tomatoes, sliced in half

½ teaspoon garlic powder

PREPARATION AND USE:

Preheat the oven to 400°F (200°C, or gas mark 6). Cover the onion slices with the lemon juice and set aside to soak. Spray a glass baking dish with a light coating of olive oil. Slice off the ends of the asparagus and line up the spears in the dish. Drizzle the olive oil over the asparagus and toss to coat. Roast for about 10 minutes.

Remove the asparagus from the oven and cut each spear into thirds. In a medium-size bowl, toss together the asparagus, artichoke hearts, and cherry tomatoes. Stir in the onion slices and their lemony marinating liquid. Sprinkle the salad with the garlic powder and toss.

YIELD: 4 servings

How it works: Packed with 135 milligrams of calcium, a medium-size artichoke is a bone support system.

Super Green Sauté

2 tablespoons (28 ml) olive oil

4 garlic cloves, minced

¼ cup (28 g) diced pecans

¼ cup (35 g) raisins

4 cups (144 g) collards, chopped, stems removed

4 cups (220 g) turnip greens, chopped

½ cup (120 ml) water

Salt and freshly ground black pepper

Sprigs of parsley, for garnish

PREPARATION AND USE:

Heat the olive oil in a large skillet over medium heat. Add the garlic and sauté for about a minute. Add the pecans, raisins, and greens and sauté for 4 to 5 minutes until the greens wilt. Pour in the water and then let it boil away. Remove from the heat, transfer to plates, add salt and pepper to taste, and garnish with parsley.

YIELD: 2 servings

How it works: These leafy greens contain a powerful calcium punch. One-half cup (95 g) of cooked collards or (72 g) turnip greens provides about 100 milligrams of calcium. Parsley, pecans, and raisins contain lesser amounts of calcium, as well as other bone-friendly nutrients. Further, leafy greens and raisins are alkaline. That's important because bones release calcium salts to neutralize excess acid in the body.

Note: Alternatively, add or substitute your favorite greens: Chinese cabbage, kale, mustard greens, dandelion greens, or purslane.

Bone-Boosting Tahini

Use this Middle Eastern staple to make hummus, add to a calcium-rich legume soup, or use in the Taratoor with Crudités (at right).

2½ cups (360 g) sesame seeds

¾ cup (175 ml) olive oil, plus more if needed

PREPARATION AND USE:

Preheat the oven to 350°F (180°C, or gas mark 4). Spread the sesame seeds on a baking sheet and toast the seeds for about 10 minutes, tossing several times to prevent scorching. Remove the seeds from the oven and let cool for 15 minutes. Place the sesame seeds and olive oil in a food processor. Blend for about 2 minutes to gain a thick but pourable consistency, adding more oil if needed. Store in an airtight container for up to three weeks.

YIELD: 2 cups (480 g)

How it works: One ounce (28 g) of roasted sesame seeds contains about 280 milligrams of calcium. Sesame seeds are high in calcium and other nutrients.

Taratoor with Crudités

Sesame seeds run on the acidic side. Temper that effect by spreading taratoor on carrots, celery sticks, sugar snap peas, and other vegetables. This traditional Middle Eastern dip combines sesame seed paste (tahini) with garlic, lemon, and water.

For the taratoor:

1 cup (240 g) Bone-Boosting Tahini (at left)

1 garlic clove, crushed

Juice of 2 lemons, plus more as needed

¼ cup (60 ml) water, plus more as needed

1 teaspoon (6 g) salt

¼ cup (15 g) chopped fresh parsley

For the crudités:

1 broccoli crown, steamed and cooled

1 cup (128 g) baby carrots

2 celery stalks, chopped

1 cup (75 g) sugar snap peas

PREPARATION AND USE:

Blend all the taratoor ingredients in a blender until smooth. Add more lemon, as needed, to reach the tangy flavor desired, and more water as needed for the desired consistency. Serve with the crudités.

YIELD: 4 appetizer servings of taratoor and veggies

How it works: With veggies, this Mediterranean dip will nourish your bones. Sesame is a calcium king and broccoli alone has 178 milligrams of calcium in 1 cup (71 g).

Soy Snack

Enjoy this dish for lunch or as an afternoon snack.

1 large apple, cored and cut into chunks

½ cup (75 g) golden raisins

½ cup (50 g) crushed almonds

1 cup (230 g) vanilla soy yogurt

Pinch of ground cinnamon

PREPARATION AND USE:

In a medium-size bowl, mix together the apple, raisins, and almonds. Blend in the yogurt and sprinkle with the cinnamon. Enjoy.

YIELD: 1 large or 2 small servings

How it works: Raisins and almonds contain calcium. In fact, 1 ounce (28 g) of almonds (20 to 25 nuts) has as much calcium as ¼ cup (60 ml) of milk. Apples and especially raisins are alkalinizing, helping bones retain calcium and reducing the risk of osteoporosis.

Pom-Tan-Chia

1 tablespoon (13 g) chia seeds

1 cup (235 ml) pomegranate juice

1 cup (235 ml) calcium-fortified tangerine juice

PREPARATION AND USE:

Place the chia seeds in a clean, wide-mouthed pint-size (475 ml) jar, pour in the juices, and stir. Cap the jar and shake until completely blended. Leave in the refrigerator for about 2 hours and then serve.

YIELD: 2 servings

How it works: One tablespoon (13 g) of chia seeds contains 65 milligrams of calcium, as well as magnesium and potassium. And pomegranate juice is a major source of antioxidants, making this a healthy anytime drink.

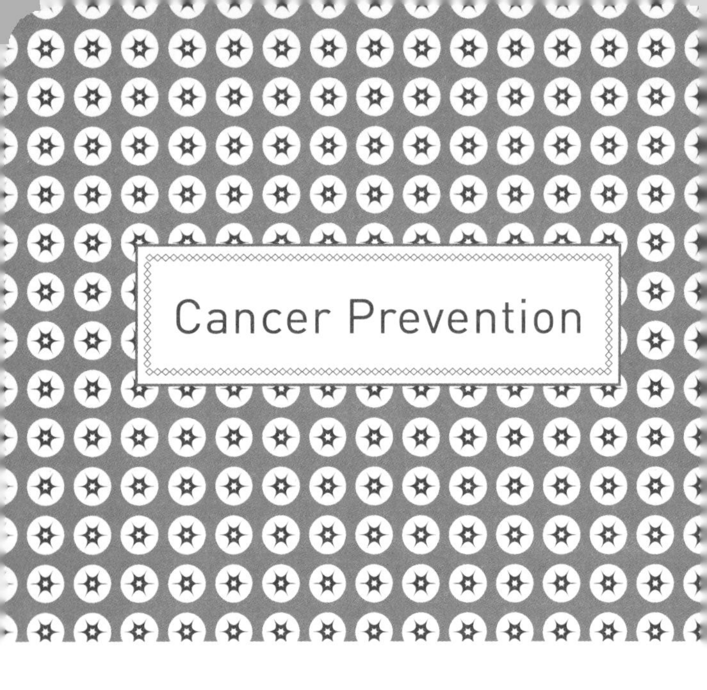

Cancer Prevention

The big C. The crab. The crustacean that scuttles in and out of nightmares. Too many of us know the touch of its claw. Cancer is the second-leading cause of death in the United States, accounting for one in four deaths. Annually, an estimated 1.6 million Americans receive a cancer diagnosis—a number that excludes skin cancers, which are so common they're not reported to cancer registries. The most common cancers involve the lung, colon, breast, and prostate; combined they cause half of all cancer deaths.

Many types of cancer are either preventable or easily treatable. In terms of lifestyle factors, scientists attribute one-third of cancers to tobacco use, one-third to diet, and one-third to environmental exposures (infectious microorganisms, ultraviolet light, radiation, pollutants, and other toxins). Physical inactivity, obesity, insufficient sleep, and alcohol are also linked to some cancers. Genetics play a significant role in only a few cancers.

Keep in mind that twenty to thirty years often elapse between the microscopic start of cancer and diagnosis of a tumor. A host of events can conspire to initiate and propagate a tumor. Furthermore, we can't completely control environmental exposures and have zero control over past exposures. What we can all do is to start now to reduce our modifiable risks. A number of organizations provide information on how to do just that: Prevent Cancer (http://preventcancer.org), the American Cancer Society (http://www.cancer.org), and the National Cancer Institute (www.cancer.gov). Authorities agree that the four most important things you can do to prevent cancer are to avoid tobacco, eat a healthy diet, exercise regularly, and get recommended screening tests.

Go Greek Salad

1 teaspoon (5 g) fresh lemon juice
4 teaspoons (20 ml) olive oil, divided
Sea salt and freshly ground black pepper
6 ounces (170 g) salmon
2 tablespoons (30 ml) red wine vinegar
1 garlic clove, crushed
3 cups (141 g) torn romaine lettuce
½ medium-size cucumber, peeled and diced
1 Roma tomato, diced
¼ cup (35 g) pitted and sliced black olives
¼ cup (40 g) diced red onion
¼ cup (38 g) crumbled feta cheese

PREPARATION AND USE:

Preheat the oven to 450°F (230°C, or gas mark 8). In a small bowl, mix together the lemon juice, 1 teaspoon (5 ml) of the olive oil, and a pinch of salt and pepper. Baste the salmon in the mixture, transfer to a roasting pan, and roast for 10 minutes.

Meanwhile, in a large bowl, whisk together remaining 3 teaspoons (15 ml) of olive oil, and the vinegar, crushed garlic, and additional salt and pepper to taste. Toss in the lettuce, cucumber, tomato, olives, and onion. Fold in the feta. Divide between two plates. Top each with 3 ounces (85 g) of roasted salmon.

YIELD: 2 servings

How it works: The Mediterranean diet is associated with a reduced risk of cancer. It's rich in a number of foods thought to protect against cancer: vegetables, fruits, grains, legumes, and olive oil, and fish as well as a moderate amount of red wine (which contains resveratrol, an anticancer substance). Plant-based diets seem to shield us from cancer.

Color Guard

Berries, cherries, and grapes make great snack foods. Add them to smoothies or top cereal, salads, and yogurt with them.

1 cup (145 g) blueberries
1 cup (155 g) pitted, sliced cherries
1 cup (150 g) grapes
1 cup (200 g) plain nonfat Greek yogurt
Drizzle of honey
¼ cup (28 g) crushed pecans or almonds

PREPARATION AND USE:

Combine the blueberries, cherries, and grapes in a large bowl. Fold in the yogurt. Drizzle with honey. Sprinkle with the nuts. Luscious!

YIELD: 4 servings

How it works: Berries, cherries, and grapes: these tasty, nutrient-dense packets owe their red, blue, and purple color to flavonoids, such as anthocyanins and proanthocyanins, which pack potent antioxidant, anti-inflammatory, and anticancer effects. Red grapes contain resveratrol, a well-known anticancer substance.

Gingered Carrots

1 tablespoon (15 ml) olive oil

3 large carrots, grated

1 teaspoon (2 g) minced fresh ginger

¼ cup (60 ml) fresh orange juice

¼ cup (35 g) golden raisins

Sea salt

Zest of ½ orange

Freshly ground black pepper

PREPARATION AND USE:

In a skillet, heat the oil over medium heat. Add the carrots. Stir in the ginger and cook for about 2 minutes. Add the juice, raisins, and salt to taste. Simmer for about 2 minutes until the carrots are tender and the juice has evaporated. Stir in the zest. Sprinkle with pepper to taste.

YIELD: 2 to 3 servings

How it works: Ginger is in the same plant family as turmeric. The anticancer research on it is less extensive, but preliminary data look promising. It reduces nausea and vomiting from many causes. Some studies show it may help people going through chemotherapy.

Good for You Garlic Dip

1 tablespoon (15 ml) olive oil

1 teaspoon (5 ml) fresh lemon juice

1 cup (200 g) plain Greek yogurt

3 to 4 garlic cloves, minced

3 tablespoons (18 g) chopped fresh mint

PREPARATION AND USE:

Whisk together the olive oil and lemon juice in a small bowl or measuring cup.

Place the yogurt in a medium-size bowl. Fold the oil mixture into the yogurt and mix thoroughly. Stir in the garlic and mint. Refrigerate and serve.

YIELD: 4 appetizer servings as a dip

How it works: As noted earlier, garlic has several actions that defend against cancer.

Quick Quinoa

1 cup (235 ml) almond milk

Pinch of salt

1 cup (173 g) uncooked quinoa

1 teaspoon (2 g) ground cinnamon

2 tablespoons (18 g) golden raisins

2 tablespoons (19 g) blueberries

1 tablespoon (20 g) honey

1 tablespoon (15 g) yogurt

2 tablespoons (15 g) crushed walnuts

PREPARATION AND USE:

Pour the almond milk into a saucepan and stir in the salt, quinoa, and cinnamon. Heat the quinoa mixture over medium-low heat, stirring in the raisins and blueberries. Continue stirring until the grain has soaked up the liquid and the raisins and blueberries plump up, about 10 minutes. Add the honey. Divide between two bowls, topped with the yogurt and crushed walnuts.

YIELD: 2 servings

How it works: In addition to providing vitamins and minerals, quinoa (which is a seed) and whole grains are high in complex carbohydrates, which provide fiber and release their sugars relatively slowly into the bloodstream. Refined carbohydrates lack fiber and lead to spikes in blood sugar, insulin, and insulinlike growth factors, which can stimulate tumor growth. Fiber-rich diets seem to protect against colon cancer. Fiber may help bind to potentially cancer-causing substances in the bowel, thus preventing their absorption into the bloodstream.

Nutty Flax Breakfast

½ cup (56 g) flaxseed meal

½ cup (120 ml) almond milk

¼ cup (38 g) diced apple

¼ cup (30 g) crushed walnuts

1 tablespoon (15 g) Greek yogurt

Pinch of ground cinnamon

PREPARATION AND USE:

Mix together the flaxseeds, almond milk, apple, and walnuts in a microwave-safe glass bowl. Microwave on high for 30 seconds, stir, and heat for 30 seconds more. Remove from the microwave. Top with the yogurt and cinnamon.

YIELD: 1 to 2 servings

How it works: Seeds and nuts contain vitamins, minerals, healthy fats, and fiber. Greater consumption correlates with a reduced risk of certain cancers, particularly colon cancer. Flaxseeds, sesame seeds, sunflower seeds, and pumpkin contain lignans, which our intestinal bacteria can convert into phytoestrogens. Flaxseeds, the richest source of lignans, inhibit the growth of breast, colon, and prostate cancer. Regular consumption of pumpkin and sunflower seeds has been linked with a reduced risk of breast cancer. Walnuts also inhibit colon and breast cancer.

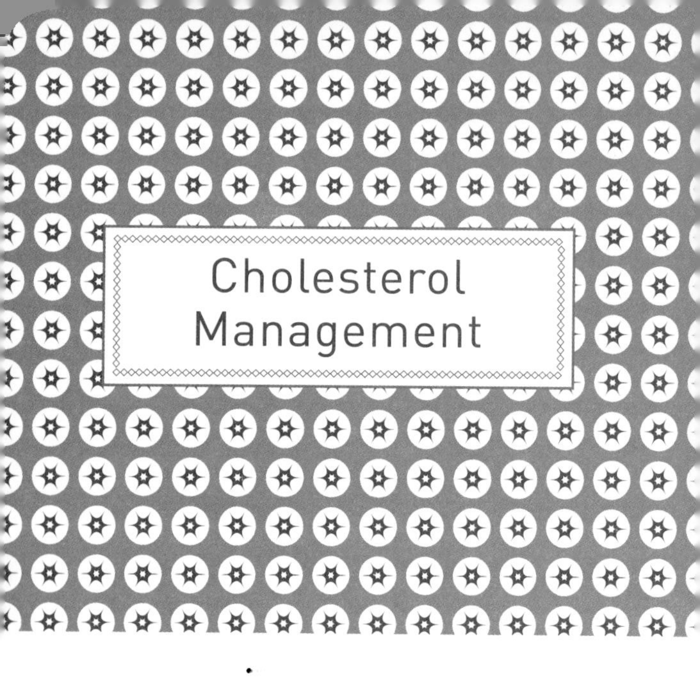

Cholesterol gets a bad rap. You know—the stuff that gums up the arteries and causes heart disease. But this waxy, much-maligned molecule is also essential. Our body requires cholesterol to form the outer layer of cells, make vitamin D, and produce hormones, such as estrogen, progesterone, and testosterone. It's so important that our livers manufacture plenty of it, regardless of whether we get it in such foods as meat, poultry, fish, eggs, and dairy.

But, yes, too much cholesterol is harmful. High cholesterol is a big risk factor for atherosclerosis, a disease in which cholesterol, fat, calcium, and other substances narrow and harden the arteries and lead to reduced blood flow. The result is heart attack, stroke, and vascular disease. Atherosclerosis is the leading cause of death in people over age forty-five. For most Americans, it takes root in childhood and progresses with each passing year. Genetics influence blood levels. Some people, no matter how healthy their lifestyle, have elevated levels.

Cholesterol travels in a package called a lipoprotein. These little protein-cholesterol tugboats transport several types of cholesterol, including low-density, high-density, very low-density, and other fats, through the blood. The lower the density, the greater the fatty freight. That's why low-density lipoprotein (LDL) and very-low-density lipoprotein (VLDL) are "bad," and high-density lipoprotein (HDL), which can pick up excess cholesterol and carry it to the liver for elimination, is "good." Further, LDL cholesterol becomes toxic to our cells when oxidized, a process akin to butter going rancid. Oxidized cholesterol causes free radical damage and promotes atherosclerosis. So your goals are to keep VLDL and LDL cholesterol within normal limits. Fortunately, nature provides a host of plants that do just that.

RECIPES TO SUPPORT HEALTHY CHOLESTEROL LEVELS

Mom's Oatmeal

1 cup (235 ml) water

½ cup (40 g) regular or quick-cooking (not instant) rolled oats

Pinch of salt

½ cup (75 g) diced apple

2 tablespoons (15 g) sliced or chopped walnuts

Honey (optional)

1 teaspoon (2 g) ground cinnamon

PREPARATION AND USE:

Combine the water, oats, and salt in a microwave-safe bowl. Microwave on high for 1 minute and then stir in the apple, walnuts, and cinnamon. Microwave for another minute. Remove from the microwave. Taste it before adding honey. (The apple provides natural sweetness.) Enjoy while still piping hot.

YIELD: 1 serving

How it works: Oatmeal contains soluble fiber, which reduces the absorption of dietary cholesterol from the intestines into the blood. Some research shows that cinnamon can reduce cholesterol. Apples contain pectin and flavonoids that both lower cholesterol. Walnuts also lower cholesterol.

Psyllium Smoothie

¼ cup (38 g) strawberries

¼ cup (38 g) blueberries

½ banana

1 cup (235 ml) water

3 ice cubes (optional)

1½ teaspoons (10 g) honey (optional)

1 teaspoon (6 g) psyllium husks

PREPARATION AND USE:

Place the fruits in a blender. Add the water, ice cubes (if desired), honey, and psyllium and blend until smooth. Enjoy!

YIELD: 1 serving

How it works: Fiber-rich psyllium seed husks, when mixed with water, form a gel that binds cholesterol in the intestine, thereby reducing its absorption into the blood. It also increases the elimination of cholesterol from the body. These fruits provide fiber and antioxidants.

Artichokes and Garlic Dip

1 cup (235 ml) olive oil

1 garlic clove, crushed

Salt and freshly ground black pepper

2 artichokes

¼ cup (60 ml) water

PREPARATION AND USE:

Pour the olive oil into a small bowl. Mix in the garlic. Stir in salt and pepper to taste. On a cutting board, cut the artichoke stems to 1 inch (2.5 cm) long. Snip off the sharp tips of the petals. Slice each one in half lengthwise. Scoop out the prickly "choke" inside. Fill a microwave-safe dish with the water. Lay out the four artichoke halves, cut side down, and cover with waxed paper or a lid. Microwave on HIGH until tender, about 10 minutes. Let stand for 1 to 2 minutes to cool. Pull off the leaves and dip the fleshy part into the olive oil mixture.

YIELD: 2 servings

How it works: Artichokes are shown to reduce LDL cholesterol. Some studies indicate that garlic reduces LDL cholesterol. It protects LDL from oxidation, discourages blood clots from forming within the arteries, modestly lowers blood pressure, helps maintain the elasticity of arteries, and slows the development of atherosclerosis.

Warning: Stop taking garlic supplements two weeks before surgery. If you're taking blood-thinning medication such as warfarin (Coumadin), talk to your doctor first before adding garlic supplements or raw garlic to your diet. Garlic could potentially increase the action of the medication.

Beneficial Barley Soup

3 cups (710 ml) water

½ cup (92 g) uncooked barley

1 tablespoon (15 ml) olive oil

1 onion, finely chopped

1 teaspoon (3 g) diced garlic

½ cup (35 g) sliced mushrooms

2 tablespoons (32 g) miso paste

Pinch of freshly ground black pepper

1 cup (248 g) cubed tofu (optional)

PREPARATION AND USE:

In a large pot, combine the water and barley. Bring to a boil, lower the heat, and simmer on low heat for 30 minutes. In a separate pan, combine the olive oil, onion, garlic, and mushrooms and sauté over medium heat until tender, about 5 minutes. Add the miso paste and pepper to the sauté pan. Then add the tofu, if using, and continue cooking the mixture for an additional 2 minutes. Pour the sautéed mixture into the barley pot. Stir well. Ladle the mixture among four plates.

YIELD: 4 servings

How it works: Barley is made of the viscous, or soluble, fiber, which helps keep cholesterol from absorbing into the blood. Studies show that replacing animal protein with soy foods can lower LDL cholesterol and blood pressure, among other benefits.

Hummus Dip with Celery Sticks

1 can (14 ounces, or 400 g) chickpeas, drained and rinsed

2/3 cup (153 g) plain low-fat yogurt

I garlic clove, chopped

Pinch of paprika, plus more if desired

Pinch of ground cumin

Juice of ½ lemon

Olives, sliced cucumbers, and tomatoes, for garnish

Celery sticks

PREPARATION AND USE:

Place the chickpeas, yogurt, and garlic in a blender and blend until smooth. Add the paprika, cumin, and lemon juice and blend once more until smooth. Pour the hummus into a serving dish and garnish with the olives, cucumbers, and tomatoes. Add additional paprika, if desired. Serve with celery sticks.

YIELD: 4 to 6 servings

How it works: Chickpeas are a rich source of soluble fiber, keeping cholesterol from absorbing into the blood. They also provide omega-3 fats, potassium, and manganese.

Recipe Variation: Add red bell pepper sticks as a garnish, or substitute for the celery.

Wholly Guacamole

3 avocados, peeled, pitted, and mashed

Juice of 1 lime

1 teaspoon (6 g) salt

½ cup (80 g) diced onion

3 tablespoons (3 g) chopped fresh cilantro

2 small tomatoes, diced

1 teaspoon (3 g) minced garlic

Pinch of cayenne

½ teaspoon hot sauce (optional)

PREPARATION AND USE:

In a medium-size bowl, mash the avocados with the lime juice and salt. Mix in the onion, cilantro, tomatoes, and garlic. Stir in the cayenne and hot sauce, if using. Serve immediately.

YIELD: 6 servings

How it works: tudies show that avocado, an excellent source of soluble fiber, has 15 grams of heart-healthy unsaturated fat, helps reduce LDL, and may increase HDL cholesterol. Lab studies show that cayenne lowers cholesterol and protects it from oxidation.

Recipe Variation: Use ½ cup (130 g) of salsa instead of the cilantro, tomatoes, and garlic.

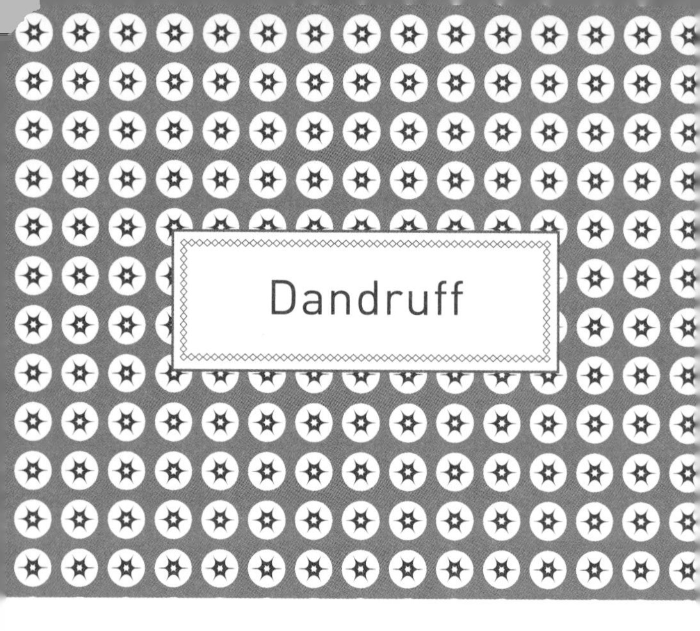

You win some, you lose some. This principle holds true not only for economics but for human biology. For example, just as new cells perpetually form at the base of the skin and scalp, old cells slough off the surface. These cells comprise much of the dust in your house.

For some reason, we have a social stigma against visible accumulations of dead skin cells caught in our hair or dusting the shoulders of our clothes. In truth, it's all relative. Some people simply have more exuberant cell turnover, which makes the process more noticeable. In fact, dandruff affects half of us.

Dandruff can also cause itching and redness of the scalp. Heat can worsen the condition. Men have it more often than women. For many people, the scalp becomes less flaky with age.

Seborrheic dermatitis causes more severe dandruff. The affected skin and scalp becomes inflamed, very flaky, and greasy looking. Cradle cap in infants is one form of seborrheic dermatitis. Other disorders—psoriasis, eczema, fungal skin infection, and head lice—can cause scalp flakiness. A particular fungus (*Malassezia*) has now been associated with dandruff, seborrheic dermatitis, and cradle cap. It seems to thrive on excretions from the scalp's oil glands.

Sesame Asparagus

1 bunch asparagus, thick ends removed

1 tablespoon (15 ml) sesame oil

Freshly ground black pepper

1 teaspoon (3 g) sesame seeds

PREPARATION AND USE:

Preheat the oven to 450°F (230°C, or gas mark 8). On a baking sheet, toss the asparagus spears with the sesame oil. Sprinkle with pepper to taste. Roast the asparagus for 5 minutes and then turn the spears and sprinkle with the sesame seeds. Roast for 5 minutes more until the asparagus is tender and just browned. Serve immediately.

YIELD: 2 servings

How it works: Low body levels of zinc and certain B vitamins can trigger dandruff. Asparagus and sesame seeds contain both zinc and vitamin B. Leafy green vegetables are excellent delivery systems for these important nutrients, as well as nuts and seeds, including pine nuts, pecans, and pumpkin seeds.

Tea Tree Scalp Treatment

2 to 3 drops tea tree essential oil

¼ cup (60 ml) flaxseed oil

PREPARATION AND USE:

Drop the tea tree essential oil into the flaxseed oil and blend. Apply the mixture liberally to your scalp before bedtime. Wrap your head in a clean towel or cover your pillow with the towel to protect it. In the morning, shampoo and rinse your scalp thoroughly.

YIELD: 1 application

How it works: Tea tree oil has antifungal properties. Flaxseed oil contains omega-3 fatty acids, which reduce inflammation that can accompany dandruff. If you have the type of dandruff caused by dry skin, the oil may help.

LIFESTYLE TIP

If your dandruff appeared after you tried a new shampoo, switch to another, milder product—perhaps a fragrance-free, hypoallergenic shampoo. The same goes for other hair products. They can either irritate the scalp or lead to a buildup of oil. Hair dyes and permanents can be very irritating.

Rosemary Scalp Wash

1 cup (235 ml) apple cider vinegar

2 tablespoons (3 g) fresh rosemary leaves

PREPARATION AND USE:

Place the vinegar in a small pan and heat until nearly boiling. Remove from the heat, stir in the rosemary, cover the pan, and steep for 10 minutes. Strain the mixture and discard the herbs. Pour into a clean empty jar or bottle to store. After every shampoo, mix ¼ cup (60 ml) of the solution with 2 cups (475 ml) of water. Use it to rinse your scalp thoroughly.

YIELD: 4 applications

How it works: Vinegar contains acetic acid, which is antifungal. Rosemary is an excellent antibacterial and antifungal agent.

Fact or Myth?

DRY SKIN CAUSES DANDRUFF.

That depends. In seborrheic dermatitis, the skin and scalp are oily and the oils can favor the growth of a fungus called *Malassezia*. Frequent shampooing can improve dandruff but could worsen dry scalp. However, dry skin and scalp account for the fact that some people have flakier scalps in winter.

Tea Tree Oil Shampoo

¼ cup (60 ml) liquid castile soap

¼ cup (60 ml) water

½ teaspoon olive or flaxseed oil

10 to 20 drops tea tree essential oil

PREPARATION AND USE:

Place all the ingredients in a sizeable, clean squeeze bottle with a secure top. Cap and shake to combine. Part your hair in small sections. Dab the shampoo onto one small area at a time. Massage the shampoo into your scalp. Rinse.

YIELD: 4 to 6 applications

How it works: Tea tree oil is active against some species of *Malassezia*, the fungus associated with dandruff and seborrheic dermatitis. One study found that a shampoo containing 5 percent tea tree oil significantly improved dandruff relative to a placebo. Although this study did not reveal any side effects, some people are allergic to the essential oil of this plant. If this shampoo irritates your scalp, stop using it.

Note: You can also use this mild mixture as a general skin wash.

Yogurt Boost

1 cup (230 g) plain yogurt

1 tablespoon (15 ml) fresh lemon juice

PREPARATION AND USE:

In a small bowl, mix the yogurt and lemon juice. Thoroughly massage the yogurt mixture into your scalp. Cover your scalp with a shower cap or warm towel for about 30 minutes. Remove the wrap and shampoo.

YIELD: 1 application

How it works: If a case of dandruff is caused by a fungal infection, yogurt can help fight it. It contains friendly bacteria that discourage fungal infections such as Malassezia. The citric acid in lemon juice is also antifungal.

Cradle Cap Relief

Pure castile liquid soap

Mineral oil (optional)

PREPARATION AND USE:

Gently massage your infant's scalp with your fingers to help circulation and loosen scaly patches. Shampoo with the castile soap, rinsing the head thoroughly. Do this daily until the scaly patches disappear; then shampoo twice weekly. If your child has a head of hair, brush it with a clean, soft brush after each shampoo and several times during the day.

For stubborn scales: To help loosen especially stubborn scales, put mineral oil on your fingertips and massage it into your baby's scalp. Wrap a warm, wet cloth around your child's head for about an hour. (Alternate two cloths, changing one cloth for a warm cloth each time it starts to cool; you must keep the wrap warm to maintain the baby's body heat.)

YIELD: Daily application until the scales disappear

How it works: Gentle massage increases circulation for smooth skin and also helps remove the dead, scaly skin of cradle cap. The mineral oil and warm cloth helps soften especially stubborn scales. The key ingredient in castile soap is skin-softening olive oil combined with the alkaline sodium hydroxide. It has no harsh artificial additives to irritate the baby's tender scalp.

Note: Contact your doctor if the scales continue; you may need a prescription cream.

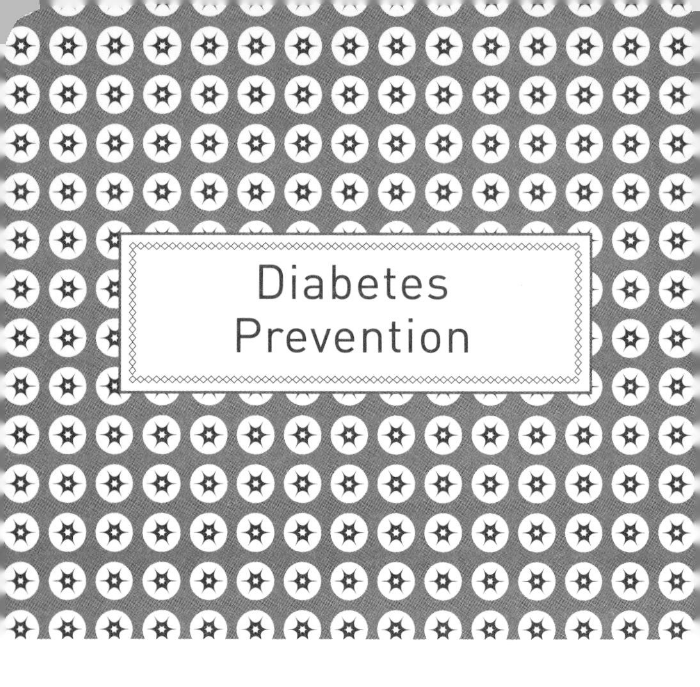

Diabetes Prevention

Worldwide, diabetes is one of the most common chronic diseases. In developed countries, diabetes has reached epidemic proportions. In the United States, it's the seventh leading cause of death. The number of Americans diagnosed with diabetes tripled between 1980 and 2010, when the number topped 20 million.

In the developing world, cases of diabetes have surged, due mainly to the importation of the Western lifestyle, particularly the combination of physical inactivity and diets high in refined grains and sugar, both of which fuel weight gain and which, in turn, promotes obesity. By 2025, experts anticipate that diabetes will afflict 246 to 380 million people worldwide.

The underlying problem in diabetes lies with insulin, a pancreatic hormone whose main function is to move glucose (sugar) from the bloodstream into liver, muscle, and fat cells. Without insulin, blood glucose levels climb, damaging many tissues, and the cells starve.

If you have diabetes, you know how important it is to control blood sugar with some combination of lifestyle modifications and medications. Consequences of chronically high blood sugar are accelerated aging of many tissues, arterial disease, heart disease and heart attack, stroke, eye disease (vision-robbing diabetic retinopathy), nerve damage, and poorly healing wounds.

Roasted Veggie Explosion

1 to 2 tablespoons (15 to 30 ml) olive oil

1 large onion, quartered

2 carrots, diced

1 red or yellow bell pepper, seeded and sliced into strips

1 bunch asparagus, woody bottoms cut off

2 beets, peeled and quartered

4 garlic cloves, peeled

¼ cup (7 g) crushed fresh rosemary

Sea salt (optional)

PREPARATION AND USE:

Preheat the oven to 400°F (200°C, or gas mark 6). Spray or brush a baking sheet with olive oil. Drizzle the olive oil over the vegetables in a bowl and toss to coat them. Spread the vegetables and garlic evenly across a baking sheet. Sprinkle with the rosemary and the sea salt to taste, if using. Roast for 15 minutes and then flip the vegetables and roast for another 10 minutes. They should be browned but not overcooked.

YIELD: 6 servings

How it works: Fruits and vegetables contain fiber, which slows absorption of dietary sugars, and many nutrients beneficial to overall health and reducing diabetes risks. The World Health Organization recommends eating at least five portions a day to prevent diabetes.

Simply Psyllium Date Loaf

1⅓ cups (120 g) gluten-free oat flour

¼ cup (28 g) flaxseed meal

2 tablespoons (36 g) psyllium powder

1½ teaspoons (7 g) baking soda

5 large eggs

¼ cup (60 ml) water

¼ cup (60 ml) coconut oil, melted

1 packet (1 g) stevia

1 tablespoon (15 g) apple cider vinegar

½ cup (89 g) chopped, seeded dates

Plain nonfat Greek yogurt

PREPARATION AND USE:

Preheat the oven to 350°F (180°F, or gas mark 4). Lightly spray a 9 x 5-inch (23 x 12.5 cm) loaf pan with canola oil. Set aside. In a large bowl, blend the flour, flaxseed meal, psyllium, and baking soda. Stir in the eggs, water, oil, stevia, and vinegar. Fold in the chopped dates. Pour into the prepared pan and bake for about 30 minutes or until the center springs back to touch. Serve warm with a dollop of yogurt.

YIELD: 1 loaf

How it works: Not only does psyllium husk prevent and correct constipation, but the fiber lowers cholesterol levels as well as blood glucose after a meal in people with type-1 and type-2 diabetes. It doesn't lower blood glucose in people who are not diabetics. Fiber helps you feel fuller, which can reduce calorie intake (a boon if you're trying to lose weight).

Flaxseed Breakfast Delight

¼ cup (28 g) flaxseed meal

¼ cup (60 ml) nonfat milk or almond milk

1 large egg

1 teaspoon (7 g) honey

¼ cup (35 g) seeded and cubed apple

1 tablespoon (7.5 g) crushed walnuts

At least 1 teaspoon (2 g) ground cinnamon (see How it works.)

PREPARATION AND USE:

Pour the flaxseed meal into a microwave-safe breakfast bowl. Stir in the milk, egg, and honey. Microwave on high for about 30 seconds. Stir the cereal, then fold in the apple and walnuts. Stir in the cinnamon. Microwave for another 30 seconds. Enjoy.

YIELD: 1 serving

How it works: Flaxseed consumption can improve some measures of disease in people with type-2 diabetes. Studies show that a compound in flaxseed called *lignan* (also called *lignin*) can improve some measures of disease in people with type-2 diabetes. Some research indicates that two species of cinnamon—Ceylon or "true" cinnamon (*Cinnamomum verum*, a.k.a. *C. zeylanicum*) or Chinese cinnamon (*Cinnamomum cassia*, or *C. aromaticum*)—lower blood glucose. Other studies have failed to find a significant effect. Because it's cheaper, Chinese cinnamon is what you'll find in most supermarkets. Look for Ceylon cinnamon in specialty stores.

Artichokes with Pepper Dip

2 garlic cloves, divided

1 cup (230 g) plain Greek yogurt

2 tablespoons (12 g) chopped fresh mint

¼ teaspoon ground cumin

1/8 teaspoon cayenne pepper

Dash of olive oil

2 artichokes

PREPARATION AND USE:

Mince one garlic clove. In a bowl, mix the yogurt, minced garlic, mint, cumin, cayenne, and olive oil. Refrigerate for at least 1 hour. While the dip is chilling, snip the sharp tips of the artichoke petals and trim the stem to about 1-inch (2.5 cm) long. Fill a large pot with about two fingers of water and drop in the other garlic clove. Place the artichokes in a steamer basket. Bring the water to a boil and steam the artichokes until you can pierce the bottom of the stems with a fork and the leaves easily pull away, about 30 minutes. Serve the artichokes warm with the cool dip.

YIELD: 2 servings

How it works: Artichoke petals and hearts are rich in fiber. Also, artichoke is related to milk thistle. Milk thistle extracts improve fast blood glucose, cholesterol levels, triglycerides, and other indicators of risk in people with type-2 diabetes. Regular consumption of cayenne and chiles may also help regulate insulin levels after a meal.

Buckwheat Blueberry Pancakes

1½ cups (180 g) buckwheat flour

1 packet (1 g) stevia

2 teaspoons (5 g) ground cinnamon

1 teaspoon (5 g) baking soda

3 tablespoons (45 ml) olive oil

2 cups (475 ml) buttermilk

1 cup (145 g) blueberries

PREPARATION AND USE:

Combine the flour, stevia, cinnamon, and baking soda in a large bowl. Drizzle in the olive oil and begin stirring. Slowly pour in the buttermilk and continue to stir, mixing only until the ingredients are just combined and still lumpy. Fold in the blueberries.

Wipe a griddle with olive oil and heat it over medium heat. Ladle the batter for the pancakes on the hot griddle. Lower the heat to medium-low, cook, and turn when the top side shows bubbles—about 2 minutes. Cook the other side for about a minute until browned.

Suitable toppings include a dollop of yogurt, a few additional fresh blueberries (or other fresh fruit), or a small amount of peanut butter. Resist the urge to smother the pancakes with syrup, honey, jam, or jelly—sugary substances that will stimulate a rapid rise in blood glucose.

YIELD: 3 to 4 servings

How it works: Buckwheat flour packs a magnesium punch. Whereas low magnesium levels seem to raise the risk of type-2 diabetes, eating a diet high in magnesium has been linked to reduced risk of developing type-2 diabetes. Studies show that just 100 milligrams put adults at a 15 percent lower risk of developing the disease. Aside from buckwheat, good sources of magnesium include spinach, beans lentils, almonds, peanuts, cashews, and wheat bran. Barley, yogurt, and halibut are other terrific sources.

LIFESTYLE TIP

Get a diabetes-fighting magnesium boost from a handful of roasted pumpkin seeds. About ¼ cup (35 g) of the seeds boasts 300 milligrams of magnesium; that's 95 percent of the recommended daily dose.

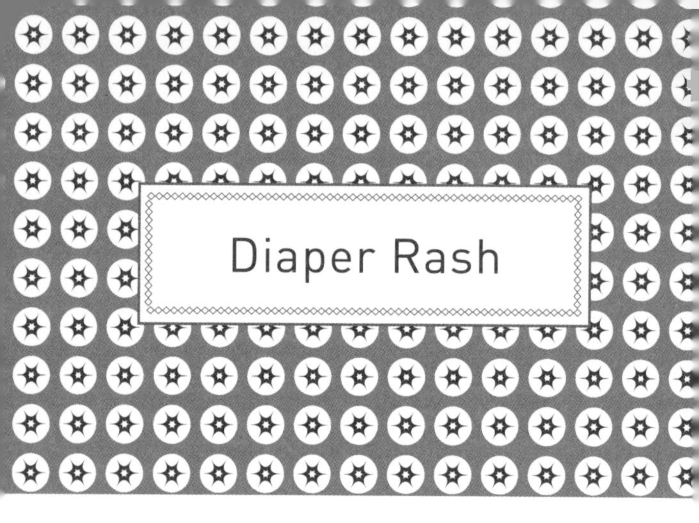

Diaper Rash

Diaper rash is so common among infants it's practically a rite of passage, along with adolescent acne and menstrual cramps. That said, the condition deserves care to prevent it from becoming severe and uncomfortable. The appearance varies from a few red, irritated spots to redness over the entire diaper area. Inflammation can make the skin look puffy and feel warm.

What causes the rash is prolonged contact between diaper contents and an infant's sensitive skin. Wastes in urine can break down to ammonia, which is very irritating. Redness can also occur in areas where the diaper chafes the skin. Another possibility is contact allergy to chemicals in commercial diaper wipes or detergents used to wash cloth diapers. There are, however, things you can do to control it.

RECIPES TO PREVENT AND TREAT DIAPER RASH

The Big Change

Warm water

Castile or other mild, nonscented soap
(Use soap only if the area is soiled.)

Commercially prepared ointment or herbal salve

PREPARATION AND USE:
Remove the wet or dirty diaper. Wash the diaper area with a cotton ball moistened in warm water. If the area is dirty, bathe with mild soap (avoid commercially prepared fragranced wipes). Gently pat dry. Apply a commercially prepared ointment or an herbal salve to the diaper area.

YIELD: 1 application

How it works: Immediate cleansing, drying, and lubricating of the diaper area with mild, natural ingredients helps keep the baby's skin fresh and supple.

Warning: Do not use powders, especially talcum powder. Inhaled talcum particles can cause lung disease. Cornstarch can worsen a yeast infection.

Fresh and Fluffy

This safe, easy wash for cloth diapers is gentle enough for baby's skin.

Hypoallergenic detergent

½ cup (120 ml) vinegar

PREPARATION AND USE:

Place soiled cloth diapers in the washing machine and add hypoallergenic detergent. Run the diapers through a full cycle, adding the vinegar to the rinse cycle. Dry as usual.

YIELD: 1 load of laundry

How it works: A hypoallergenic detergent minimizes allergic reactions. Such reactions will manifest as a rash limited to the areas the diaper contacts the skin. Vinegar is an antibacterial.

LIFESTYLE TIP

Change the diaper frequently, at least every 2 hours, until your baby begins urinating less often. Poopy diapers are hard to miss. Change these immediately, and then gently cleanse the diaper area with water or an unscented wipe.

Baby Sitz Soother

Soaking will help soothe the diaper area, especially if the skin is very raw.

2 tablespoons (28 g) baking soda

PREPARATION AND USE:

Pour warm water into a basin large enough to soak the baby's bottom. Mix in the baking soda. Soak the infant in the bath for 10 to 15 minutes. Pat your infant dry, paying attention to the diapered area. Repeat once or twice more as needed throughout the day.

YIELD: 1 application

How it works: Sitting in a warm bath is therapeutic for many babies. Cleansing the area with soothing warm water and baking soda will help counter the acidity of the affected area.

Warning: Be sure to stay with your baby constantly while he or she is in the tub.

Skin-Healing Calendula Oil

You'll find dried calendula in herb stores, some natural food stores, and through online retailers. Calendula is an easy-to-grow annual. Plant it in pots or your garden. (Make sure you're planting Calendula officinalis, *not garden marigold,* Tagetes erecta, *or* T. patula*).*

1 cup (25.5 g) dried calendula flowers

1½ cups (355 ml) oil (e.g., almond, apricot, or olive), plus more as needed

PREPARATION AND USE:

If the flower heads are whole, grind in a clean coffee grinder or food processor. Pour the flowers into a clean jar (pint-size [475 ml] should work well). Pour in the oil until you've covered the flowers. Stir with a wooden spoon or chopstick. Add another ½ to 1 inch (1.3 to 2.5 cm) of oil atop the herb and tightly screw on the lid. Place the jar inside a paper sack or box (to protect from ultraviolet rays). Set near a window or other warm area. Shake daily for one to two weeks. The oil will now be tinged a deep yellow. Line a strainer with cheesecloth or muslin. Strain. With clean, dry hands, wring as much oil as you can from the cloth-wrapped herbs. Feel free to massage the oil on your hands into your skin. It feels and smells wonderful! Pour the oil into a clean, dry bottle and cap tightly. Store in the refrigerator. Apply to clean skin as needed. Discard or compost the herbal matter.

YIELD: Multiple applications

How it works: Calendula has anti-inflammatory, antibacterial, antifungal, and wound-healing properties. One study showed that calendula cream improved diaper rash better than an aloe-based cream did. The oil protects the skin. However, even though calendula is antifungal, do not apply it if your baby develops a fungal infection. You don't want to apply oils, salves, and ointments that could trap in moisture, which promotes fungal growth.

Warning: Calendula is in the same plant family as ragweed, which means some people are also allergic to it. If you have a family history of allergies, apply calendula to a small patch of your baby's skin (an area that isn't already affected by diaper rash). It can take up to forty-eight hours for a skin rash to appear.

Note: If you can't wait two weeks, you can make this oil much sooner by substituting the recipe on page 93 that uses coconut oil.

C-Salve

1 cup (235 ml) calendula oil (page 90)

¼ cup (55 g) grated beeswax

PREPARATION AND USE:

Make the oil as instructed in the previous recipe. Pour the oil into a saucepan over low heat. Add the beeswax. Stir continuously until the beeswax melts, taking care not to burn the oil. Spoon a little of the mixture onto a clean plate and pop it in the freezer for a minute or two. If you like the consistency, you're ready to jar. If you want a firmer consistency, add more beeswax and melt. If you desire a less solid consistency, add more calendula oil. While the mixture is still warm, pour it into a clean glass jar or tin. Screw on the cap. The salve will soon solidify. Store in a cool place. Apply the salve as needed.

YIELD: Multiple applications

How it works: Beeswax adds a soothing, protective factor. It also turns the oil into a consistency that's less messy to apply. Do not apply if your baby has developed a fungal infection.

Calendula Butter

If you can't wait to make an herbal oil as in the calendula recipe on page 90, here's a faster method.

½ cup (120 g) virgin coconut oil

½ cup (120 g) shea butter

1 cup (25.5 g) dried calendula flowers

PREPARATION AND USE:

Fill the bottom of a double boiler with about 2 inches (5 cm) of water. Place the coconut oil and shea butter in the top of the double boiler. Heat the water below until the oils melt. Lower the heat to low. Add the calendula flowers and stir. Add more coconut oil if necessary so that the flowers are saturated and swimming in oil. Wait at least 1 hour (4 hours, if you have time), stirring frequently. You don't want to burn the oil. Remove the pot from the heat and carefully dry any water that has condensed on the bottom of the pan. (You want to avoid getting water in the oil.) Line a strainer with the muslin or cheesecloth and place over a bowl. Strain the warm oil. Fold the cloth around the herbs and with clean, dry hands, wring out as much oil as possible. Pour the liquid into a clean, dry jar and cap tightly. Discard or compost the herbal matter. Store in the refrigerator or cool cabinet. The oils will become solid again. Apply as needed.

YIELD: Multiple applications

How it works: Like calendula, coconut oil is anti-inflammatory. It also absorbs easily and protects the skin. Do not apply if your baby has developed a fungal infection.

Note: If you can't easily find shea butter, you can use only coconut oil.

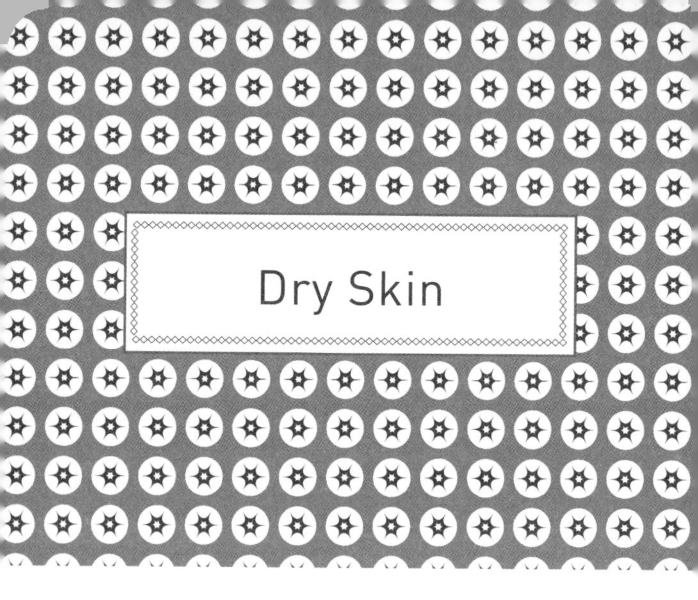

Dry Skin

For people living in arid climates, dry skin and chapped lips may be constant challenges. People with eczema and psoriasis also have dry, easily irritated skin. Age-related changes in the skin make it drier. Xerosis is the medical term for excessive dryness.

Oily substances (lipids) made by the sebaceous glands and cells within the epidermis (outer skin layer) prevent dryness. As anyone who has weathered adolescence knows, hormones make the skin oily. Specifically, androgens ("male" hormones made by both sexes) increase oil production. Heredity, humidity, age, ultraviolet light exposure, and other factors affect the relative oiliness of skin.

With age, sebaceous (oil) glands secrete less sebum. There's also a decrease in lipids made by cells within the epidermis. Decrease in skin oil makes hair less lustrous.

Essential fatty acid deficiency can also dry skin and eyes. Dry skin feels rough and looks scaly. You may also notice white flakes and patches of reddened skin. Itching is common. Don't give in to the urge to scratch, as doing so causes inflammation, breaks down the epidermis (top layer of skin), and introduces microbes into deeper layers.

The concern is more than aesthetic. Our largest organ, the skin forms a barrier against the outside world. It helps keep water from escaping and inhibits disease-causing microorganisms, ultraviolet light, and noxious chemicals from penetrating deeper. The skin's oils play an essential role in that barrier function. Some lipids discourage colonization with fungi and bacteria. Furthermore, dry skin more easily cracks, which not only hurts but also creates breeches in the barrier. Skin more easily becomes inflamed and infected.

RECIPES TO PREVENT AND TREAT DRY SKIN

Coconut Oil Rub

Extra-virgin coconut oil

PREPARATION AND USE:

Take a shower or bath. Gently pat your skin dry to remove most but not all of the water. Massage in coconut oil.

YIELD: 1 application

How it works: Pure coconut oil is an emollient, which leaves the skin soft and supple. It penetrates the skin quickly with its rich blend of saturated fatty acids, which help replace fats lost from the skin. We recommend virgin coconut oil, which is made from fresh coconut meat without the use of chemicals and high heat, thus creating a higher-quality oil.

LIFESTYLE TIP

Protect your skin from the sun. Compare the skin on your belly or buttocks with the skin on your forearm. You'll observe that ultraviolet light ages and dries the skin.

All-Natural Makeup Remover

Coconut oil (also try olive or almond oil)

PREPARATION AND USE:

Dab two to four cotton balls with enough oil for each eye and the general face. Gently swab eyes, cheeks, and lips to remove makeup. Gently wipe off the excess with a warm, damp washcloth. Rinse your face with water and pat it dry, leaving the skin damp.

YIELD: 1 application

How it works: Rather than drying out your face by washing it with soap, the coconut oil will cleanse and lubricate skin. It's especially beneficial for the eye area, where rubbing can damage sensitive skin and wrinkles are more pronounced when the skin is dry.

Skin-Salvation Salad

6 ounces (168 g) salmon

2 tablespoons (30 ml) olive oil, divided

3 cups (90 g) torn, well-rinsed spinach

1 avocado, peeled, pitted, and cut into chunks

¼ cup (25 g) pitted and sliced black olives

¼ cup (30 g) crushed walnuts

Freshly ground black pepper

2 tablespoons (30 ml) balsamic vinegar

1 tablespoon (15 ml) fresh lemon juice

PREPARATION AND USE:

Preheat the oven to broil. Brush the salmon with 1 tablespoon (15 ml) of the olive oil and place in a baking pan. Broil the salmon for 15 minutes. Meanwhile, toss together the spinach, avocado, olives, and walnuts in a large bowl. Remove the salmon from the oven when the fish flakes with a fork and allow it to cool for several minutes. Cut the salmon into chunks and toss into the salad. Sprinkle the salad with pepper to taste. In a small bowl, whisk together remaining tablespoon (15 ml) of the olive oil and the vinegar and lemon juice to make a dressing. Drizzle the dressing over the salad and give the salad a final toss.

YIELD: 3 to 4 servings

How it works: Cold-water fish, such as salmon or tuna, are high in omega-3 fatty acids. One of the symptoms of omega-3 fatty acid deficiency is dry skin and eyes. Avocado is rich in the good fats monounsaturated fatty acids and linoleic acid. One study found these fats helpful for psoriasis, although there is no research on dry skin in particular. Olives and olive oil are rich in fatty acids as are walnuts, which are packed with omega-3 fatty acids.

LIFESTYLE TIP

Eat plenty of orange and yellow veggies, such as carrots, squash, and papaya. Vitamin A deficiency, although uncommon, can cause severe dry skin, as well as other signs and symptoms. The body can convert alpha-carotene, beta-carotene, and beta-cryptoxanthin to vitamin A.

You've Got Grape Skin

6 red grapes

Water

Your moisturizer

PREPARATION AND USE:

Wash the grapes and cut them in half. Boil the water. Remove from pot from the stove and lower your head over it. Corral the vapors by draping a towel over your head. Let your face steam for 5 minutes. Gently rub the open halves of the grapes across your forehead and over your cheeks, chin, and neck. Rinse your face with cool water. Pat dry with a cool, damp washcloth. Apply your usual moisturizer.

YIELD: 1 application

How it works: Alpha-hydroxy acids (AHAs) include citric acids (in citrus fruit), glycolic acid (in cane sugar), lactic acid (in yogurt), malic acid (apples), and tartaric acid (grapes). These exfoliate, act as humectants, and increase skin pliability. Studies show that lotions containing AHAs improve dry skin.

Note: Instead of grapes, use ½ cup (115 g) of mashed papaya and paste it over your face after the steam treatment. Let it sit for 5 minutes and rinse. If your skin is sensitive, carefully apply to a small area first to check for breakout. Papaya might cause an allergic reaction in some people. Test a patch on the inside of your wrist before applying it to larger areas of skin.

Sea Salt Scrub

1 cup (236 g) sea salt

½ cup (120 ml) apricot, olive, almond, or grapeseed oil

Your moisturizer

PREPARATION AND USE:

Fully blend the salt and oil in a clean, dry jar. Set aside. Shower so that your skin is damp. While still in the shower, turn off the water, scoop out several fingerfuls (about 2 tablespoons [28 g]) of the mixture and scrub your arms and legs, avoiding any wounds or scratches. Rinse thoroughly. Pat yourself dry. Apply your regular moisturizer. Store the bottle of salt scrub in a cool area.

YIELD: About a week's worth of applications to arms and legs.

How it works: Exfoliants remove dead skin cells to reduce the scaliness of dry skin.

Warning: The oil may make the floor of the shower slippery while using this. Step carefully and rinse the floor thoroughly when finished.

Note: Alternatively, mix white or brown sugar with the oil, instead of salt.

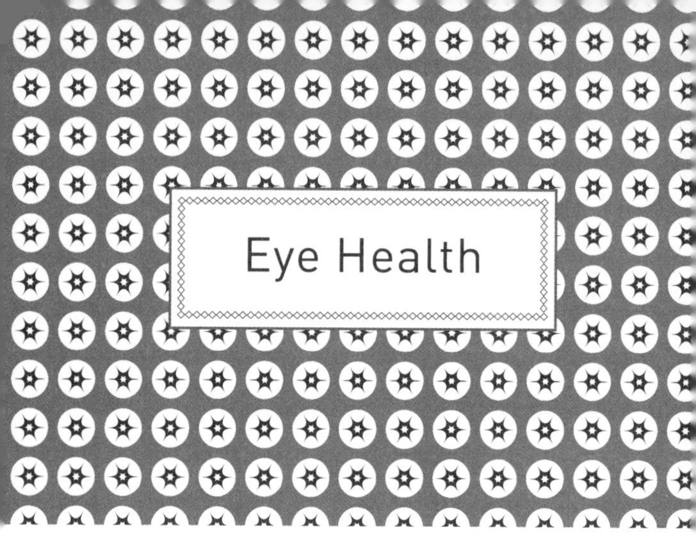

Sight is one of our most cherished senses. We navigate, read, appreciate art, admire sunsets and flowers, and connect with loved ones by gazing into these "windows of the soul."

Some eye-related conditions are relatively mild, short-lived, easily treatable, and can occur at any age. Other eye conditions are chronic. More than 14 million Americans over age twelve have a visual impairment. Excluding conditions such as nearsightedness and farsightedness (which are caused by the shape of the eye, not disease) leaves more than 3 million with the age-related diseases macular degeneration, cataracts, glaucoma, and retinopathy.

A recent survey found that the prevalence of these diseases rose more than 20 percent between 2002 and 2008—an upsurge driven in large part by an increase in diabetes. Because these conditions become more common with advancing age, the graying of the baby boomer generation only adds to the problem.

Some of the age changes in the eye happen nearly universally and, therefore, aren't considered diseases. For instance, loss of elasticity in the eye's lens makes it difficult to focus on nearby objects. We compensate with reading glasses. Other age changes reduce night vision.

Most of the other eye diseases become more common with age because they require years of wear and tear to develop. Some of them have a strong genetic component. But genetic vulnerability only rarely dictates destiny. Reducing risky lifestyle habits and improving diet can improve the odds of clear vision.

RECIPES FOR KEEPING EYES HEALTHY

Bright and Beautiful

4 medium-size yellow summer squashes, sliced lengthwise
1 red bell pepper, sliced lengthwise and seeded
1 tablespoon (15 ml) olive oil
1 red onion, sliced into rings
Freshly ground black pepper

PREPARATION AND USE:
Preheat the oven to 425°F (220°C, or gas mark 7). Lightly spray a baking sheet with the olive oil or canola cooking spray. Put the squash and bell pepper slices on the sheet. Drizzle the olive oil over the top and toss. Line up the pieces so they are not overlapping. Sprinkle the sliced onion over the top. Grind the black pepper over the vegetables. Roast for 30 minutes, turning over the veggies halfway through. Serve hot.

YIELD: 6 servings

How it works: These colorful vegetables are full of antioxidants. Furthermore, yellow, orange, and red-colored plants contain fat-soluble plant pigments called carotenoids that are, among other benefits, strong antioxidants. Two carotenoids, lutein and zeaxanthin, accumulate in the macula. Their yellow color allows them to filter out damaging blue and ultraviolet light. Higher dietary intake seems to protect against macular degeneration and cataracts. In fact, getting these nutrients from food is just as good, and possibly better, than popping them in supplement form.

Veggie-Rich Couscous

1¼ cups (219 g) uncooked couscous

½ teaspoon freshly ground black pepper

3 tablespoons (45 ml) olive oil, divided

1 yellow squash, chopped

1 yellow bell pepper, chopped

3 broccoli florets, sliced lengthwise

1 cup (235 ml) vegetable stock

2 tablespoons (8 g) chopped fresh dill

PREPARATION AND USE:

Combine couscous and peppers in a bowl. Stir in half of the olive oil to coat. Add the remaining oil to a skillet over high heat with the vegetables. Sauté them for 2 to 3 minutes until barely braised. Heat the vegetable stock to boiling in a small pan. Add the braised vegetables to the couscous and combine. Pour the boiling stock over the couscous mixture and stir. Cover the bowl with aluminum foil and steam for 5 minutes. Fluff with a fork, fold in the chopped dill, and serve.

YIELD: 4 servings

How it works: Vegetables are staples of the Mediterranean diet, which is a great example of a plant-based diet. Meals focus on fruits, vegetables, whole grains (such as couscous), nuts, olives, olive oil, and fish. Studies show that this dietary pattern, rich in vegetables, protects against cataracts and glaucoma in diabetics, a population at high risk for eye disease. Another study showed that eating at least three servings a day of antioxidant-rich vegetables reduced cataract risk.

Hail to Kale!

1 bunch of kale (about a pound [455 g]), washed, stems and ribs removed

4 teaspoons [20 ml) olive oil, divided

½ cup (120 ml) water

2 garlic cloves, minced

2 teaspoons (10 ml) vinegar

Cayenne pepper

¼ cup (28 g) crushed pecans

PREPARATION AND USE:

Chop the kale into small pieces. In a large skillet, heat 1 tablespoon (15 ml) of the olive oil over medium heat. Add the kale and toss it in the oil for about a minute. Add the water, cover, and steam over low heat for about 10 minutes. When done, push the kale to one side. To the open area of the skillet, add the final teaspoon (5 ml) of oil and the garlic, cooking the garlic for about 40 seconds. Remove the skillet from the heat and stir the garlic and kale together. Mix in the vinegar. Sprinkle the kale with cayenne pepper to taste and toss in the pecans. Serve warm.

YIELD: 4 servings

How it works: Green leafy vegetables are important dietary sources of lutein. Kale tops the list of foods rich in lutein and zeaxanthin. Other good sources include other green leafy vegetables (spinach, Swiss chard, collards, mustard, beet and turnip greens, and romaine lettuce), winter squash, okra, broccoli, Brussels sprouts, green peas, pumpkin, carrots, and tangerines.

Tuna Twice, Curried

Use the other two steaks in the previous recipe to top lunchtime salads or in this yummy curried tuna salad mix on whole wheat crackers with a side of sliced red peppers.

2 tuna steaks, cooked (4 ounces, or 115 g)
2 tablespoons (30 g) plain low-fat Greek yogurt
2 tablespoons (22 g) brown mustard
1 teaspoon (5 g) prepared horseradish
3 tablespoons (45 ml) pickle juice
2 tablespoons (18 g) chopped pickle
1 tablespoon (10 g) minced onion
Curry powder

PREPARATION AND USE:

Cut the tuna into small chunks and place in a bowl. Mash in the yogurt, mustard, horseradish, and pickle juice. Fold in the pickle and onion. Sprinkle in curry powder to taste. Serve.

YIELD: 2 servings

How it works: Tuna's omega-3 fatty acids promote eye health as noted above. Turmeric, the key spice in curry, contains curcumin, which creates the yellow color and packs a powerful anti-inflammatory and antioxidant punch. Curcumin shows promise in combating glaucoma and macular degeneration. The antioxidant-rich red peppers add eye-health benefits.

Blueberry-Bilberry Waffle Toss

Research shows that bilberry extracts defend against cataracts and glaucoma and improve diabetic and hypertensive retinopathy.

¼ cup (38 g) blueberries

¼ cup (30 g) dried bilberries (If bilberries are not available, double the blueberries to total ½ cup [75 g].)

¼ cup (39 g) sliced, pitted cherries or strawberries

¼ teaspoon ground nutmeg

¼ teaspoon ground cinnamon

4 whole-grain toaster-style waffles

1 cup (230 g) low-fat Greek yogurt

PREPARATION AND USE:

Combine the fruit in a bowl, sprinkle with the spices, and toss. Place a nonstick skillet over medium-high heat. Pour in the fruit and toss continuously for about a minute to soften. Toast the waffles. Top each waffle with a dollop of yogurt. Cover the yogurt with the fruit (the fruit will be especially sweet because the quick cooking brings out their flavor).

YIELD: 2 to 4 Servings

How it works: Many blue-, purple-, and ruby-colored berries owe their color to a type of flavonoid called anthocyanins, a potent antioxidant and blood-vessel strengthener. Top sources include bilberries, blackberries, blueberries, huckleberries, pomegranates, black currants, cherries, elderberries, cranberries, and eggplants. The blueberry is related to the bilberry, which is native to Europe. Whereas blueberries' inner flesh is white, bilberries' is blue, making them higher in anthocyanins. Anthocyanins protect the retina (light-sensitive layer at the back of the eye) and help regenerate a pigment in the eye responsible for seeing under low illumination. Although initial studies suggested the bilberries improved night vision, more recent trials didn't pan out. Volunteers in these studies were young and had normal night vision. We don't yet know whether bilberry might help elders with deteriorating night vision. Bilberries, however, have shown promise in improving retinopathy (disease of the retina) caused by diabetes and high blood pressure.

Note: Unless you live in Europe, you probably won't find fresh bilberries. You can order them dried from herbal retailers. The blueberry is an accessible runner-up for eye health.

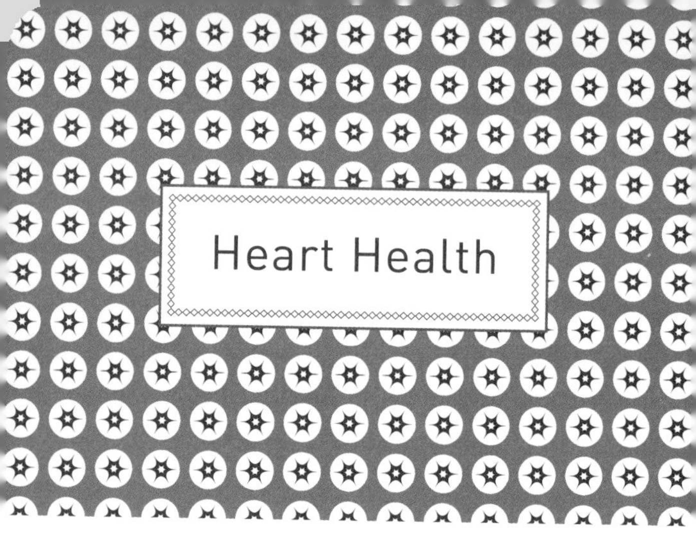

Heart Health

Here's the bad news: Heart disease is the number one killer in America. Now for the good news: Heart disease is largely preventable—and small steps can make a big difference to your heart health. For example, even one hour of physical activity a week in an otherwise sedentary lifestyle is a good start.

The most common heart problem is coronary artery disease (also called coronary heart disease). The coronary arteries encircle the heart, supplying it with oxygen and nutrients and carrying away wastes. Like other arteries in the body, the coronary arteries can become diseased. The usual culprit is atherosclerosis, a condition in which fatty material is deposited within the arterial walls. Atherosclerosis impairs circulation to the heart and other tissues in the body and increases blood pressure. The heart now has to pump blood through narrowed, rigid arteries. It's hard work. Like any other overused muscle, the heart hypertrophies, or thickens. Eventually, it starts to give out, leading to congestive heart failure.

The sooner you take steps to protect your heart the better. Here are some ways to have a healthier heart:

- Steer clear of tobacco smoke.
- Get moving. Sedentary behavior increases heart disease risk.
- Eat foods that support heart health. Make "strive for five"—five servings of fruit and vegetables daily—your mantra. Consume fish twice a week. If you eat meat, choose lean cuts. Avoid fried foods and processed foods (most of which are high in sugar and unhealthy fats).
- Cut down on sweets.
- Keep to a healthy weight.
- Get enough sleep.
- Keep regular appointments with your doctor to make sure your blood pressure and cholesterol within normal limits

Go Fish! Quick Salmon Salad Spread

1 can salmon, drained (6 ounces, or 168 g)

2 tablespoons (20 g) minced red onion

1 tablespoon (15 ml) fresh lemon juice

1½ teaspoons (7.5 ml) olive oil

1/8 teaspoon freshly ground black pepper

2 tablespoons (30 g) low-fat cream cheese

4 large, whole-grain crackers

4 slices tomato

1 large romaine lettuce leaf, cut in half

PREPARATION AND USE:

In a medium-size bowl, combine the salmon, onion, lemon juice, oil, and pepper. Spread the cream cheese on each cracker. Spread the salmon mixture over the cream cheese. Top with tomato and lettuce.

YIELD: 2 servings

How it works: Cold-water fish, such as salmon, mackerel, sardines, and herring, contain heart healthy omega-3 fatty acids called DHA (docosahaenoic acid) and EPA (eicosapentaenoic acid). These so-called fish oils decrease inflammation and triglycerides, raise HDL (good) cholesterol, discourage blood from clotting within the arteries, inhibit progression of atherosclerosis, stabilize heart rhythm to reduce the risk of sudden cardiac death, and possibly lower blood pressure.

Resveratrol-Rich Mulled Wine

1 bottle (1.5 L) red wine

1 tablespoon (7 g) ground cinnamon

1½ teaspoons (3 g) ground cloves

1½ teaspoons (3 g) ground ginger

1½ teaspoons (3 g) ground nutmeg

Grated zest of 1 lemon

Grated zest of 1 orange (Slice and reserve the orange.)

Honey

Extra ground cinnamon, for sprinkling

PREPARATION AND USE:

Place a large pot over low heat. Pour in the wine. Combine the spices and citrus zest in a tea satchel or tie into a piece of cheesecloth and place in the pan. Heat for 30 minutes. Stir in honey to taste. Pour the wine through a strainer into a decanter. Pour into mugs and top with a sprinkling of cinnamon and a slice from the zested orange.

YIELD: About 8 mugs

How it works: Red grapes, purple grape juice, and red wine contain resveratrol and other flavonoids that protect the heart and blood vessels. Some studies have linked moderate alcohol consumption with cardiovascular benefits. However, high amounts of alcohol damage the heart.

Warning: Women should drink no more than one 5-ounce (150 ml) glass of wine; and for men, the limit is two 5-ounce (150 ml) glasses. Always ask your doctor about the limit for you.

Nut-ritious Salad

I add a mixture of almonds, pecans, and Brazil nuts to this for an extra boost of heart-healthy omega-3s. ~ BHS

1 cup (55 g) torn lettuce or salad mix

1 tangerine, seeded and separated into sections

¼ cup (30 g) crushed walnuts

2 tablespoons (14 g) flaxseed meal

¼ cup (60 ml) olive oil

¼ cup (60 ml) balsamic vinegar

PREPARATION AND USE:

In a bowl, combine the lettuce, tangerine sections, and walnuts. Sprinkle in the flaxseeds. Toss. Shake together oil and vinegar and sprinkle over the top. If not using all the dressing, store the rest in the refrigerator.

YIELD: 1 main course serving or 2 side salad servings

How it works: Walnuts are rich in omega-3 fatty acids and polyphenols (compounds with potent antioxidant and anti-inflammatory effects). Studies have linked consumption of walnuts with a reduced risk of cardiovascular disease. These nuts seem to lower blood cholesterol, reduce inflammation, and improve arterial function. They also have omega-3 fatty acids, as do flaxseeds (and flaxseed oil). The body converts the fatty acids in plants to EPA and DHA.

Do the Chai-Chai

In Ayurvedic medicine, chai spices are considered sattvic: they calm, vitalize, and increase clarity, all key to less stress and heart health.

1 cup (235 ml) water

1 tea bag Darjeeling or other preferred tea

½ teaspoon ground cinnamon

½ teaspoon ground ginger

3 each: cardamom seeds, whole cloves, peppercorns

1 teaspoon (7 g) honey, or 1 packet (1 g) stevia

¼ cup (60 ml) nonfat milk

PREPARATION AND USE:

Put the water in a small saucepan. Add the tea bag, spices, and sweetener. Bring to a boil and simmer for 2 minutes. Add the milk. Strain the tea into a teapot.

YIELD: 1 serving

How it works: Studies have linked regular consumption of green and black tea with a lower risk of cardiovascular disease. Consumption of tea, whether it's green or black, benefits the heart and arteries. Cardamom, ginger, and cloves decrease platelet stickiness. (Platelets are blood cell fragments that form clots. When blood clots develop within the coronary arteries or brain arteries, heart attack or stroke develops.) Pepper contains piperine, which lab studies show lowers blood pressure. In one study involving the addition of dietary cinnamon in people with diabetes, cinnamon decreased blood levels of glucose (sugar) and cholesterol, both of which are risk factors for heart disease. In a subsequent study, only glucose significantly declined.

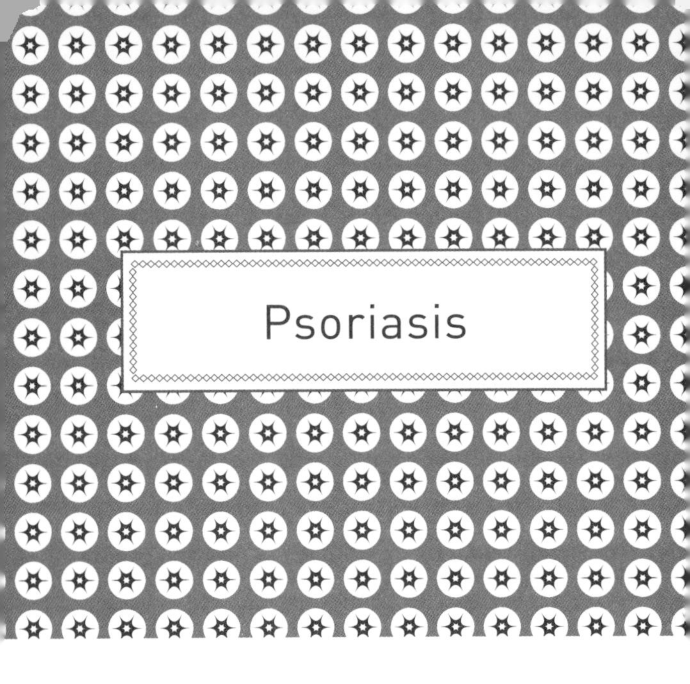

Psoriasis

Psoriasis is a common, chronic skin condition. The immune system generates inflammation in the skin, as well as other bodily tissues. Inflammatory chemicals spur excessive multiplication of cells in the epidermis, or outer layer of skin. Normally, new cells continually form at the base of the epidermis and move to the top, where they slough off. In psoriasis, new cell production outpaces the shedding of old cells, leading to a pileup at the surface, like an unraked lawn in autumn.

These raised patches on the skin are called plaques. The pink or red patches are sometimes itchy and topped by silvery scales. There may be one patch or many. The scalp, elbows, buttocks, and knees are most commonly affected.

Although scientists have yet to pinpoint the exact cause, both genetic and environmental factors contribute to psoriasis. Although often chronic, psoriasis waxes and wanes. Triggers include stress, physical trauma (a cut, scratch, or scrape), sunburn, tobacco smoke, infections, low blood calcium levels, some medications, and perhaps diet. Some people with psoriasis are sensitive to gluten, a protein found in wheat and other grains, and a gluten-free diet seems to help them. Consult your doctor about the role diet may play in treating psoriasis.

Inflammation can affect other parts of the body. Fingernails and toenails may become pitted and discolored. Up to 10 percent of people with skin plaques develop psoriatic arthritis, a potentially debilitating condition requiring strong medications.

Mega Omega Salmon Salad

1 pound (455 g) salmon fillet or 4 salmon steaks, preferably wild

¼ cup (60 ml) fresh lemon juice

Salt and freshly ground black pepper

2 onions, diced

1 tablespoon (15 ml) olive oil

1 tablespoon (15 ml) balsamic vinegar

1 tablespoon (4 g) minced fresh dill

Sliced cucumber, capers, and fresh parsley, for garnish

PREPARATION AND USE:

Preheat the oven to 375°F (190°C, or gas mark 5). Place the salmon in a baking dish and brush the fish with the lemon juice. Sprinkle with salt and pepper. Bake for 20 minutes. Remove from the oven and let cool. Skin and debone the fish, and then slice the salmon into chunks and toss into a large bowl along with the onion. In a separate bowl, combine the oil, vinegar, and dill. Pour over the salmon chunks and toss. Add salt and pepper to taste. Refrigerate for 20 minutes. Garnish the final dish with cucumbers, capers, and parsley. Serve chilled.

YIELD: 4 servings

How it works: Salmon is high in omega-3 fatty acids, which have anti-inflammatory effects. The eicosapentaenoic acid (EPA) in fish oil may be particularly valuable. A few studies have shown benefits from oral and topical preparations of EPA.

Calming Capsaicin Rub

1 chile pepper

PREPARATION AND USE:

Wash the pepper. Cut lengthwise and remove the seeds. Rub a small piece over psoriatic skin. Be sure to wash your hands thoroughly with soap and water before touching your eyes, nose, genitals, or any cuts or scrapes.

YIELD: 1 application

How it works: Chile peppers produce the hot-tasting powder cayenne. Capsaicin is a key ingredient in cayenne. Capsaicin depletes substance P, a chemical involved in pain transmission. Substance P also contributes to itching. Frequent applications of capsaicin cream can reduce itching associated with psoriasis.

Warning: With either product, expect to feel temporary heat before itching decreases.

Note: Alternatively, buy a commercially prepared cream that contains capsaicin.

Chamomile Compress

1 cup (235 ml) water

1 German chamomile tea bag

PREPARATION AND USE:

Boil the water and drop in the tea bag. Remove from the heat and let cool. Remove the tea bag. Dunk a piece of gauze or clean cloth into the tea. Apply to the affected area.

YIELD: 1 application

How it works: German chamomile (*Matricaria recutita*) reduces inflammation, inhibits bacteria, and speeds wound healing.

Warning: If you're allergic to chamomile, skip this recipe. If you're allergic to ragweed or other plants in the same family, first try this recipe on a small test area, wait twenty-four hours, and stop if inflammation occurs.

Turmeric and Aloe Paste

1 tablespoon (7 g) ground turmeric

Aloe Vera gel

PREPARATION AND USE:

Put the turmeric in a small bowl. Mix in just enough aloe gel to make a paste. Dot onto patches of the inflamed skin. Let the paste dry for about 15 minutes. Wash away.

YIELD: 1 application

How it works: Turmeric contains the potent anti-inflammatory chemical curcumin. Lab studies show that it has antipsoriasis activity when used both externally and internally. Anecdotal reports suggest that it reduces symptoms when taken internally through capsules or added as a spice to food. Aloe has its own benefits and can help move other chemicals across the skin.

Warning: Some people develop contact dermatitis (skin rash) from turmeric. Try a small test patch first and wait several hours before applying again. Also, wear old clothing when using this treatment! Turmeric, which is also used as a textile dye, can stain clothes and temporarily yellow your skin.

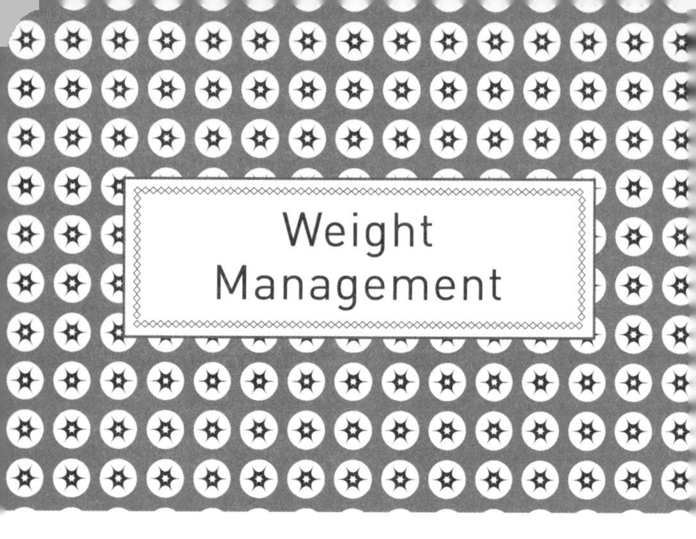

Weight Management

Which would you rather have: (a) the Fountain of Youth or (b) a body like Halle Berry (or Daniel Craig, if you're a guy)? It's a tough choice. We're betting that most red-blooded Americans would go with (b). Here's why: One, humans like instant gratification. Two, being lean and healthy correlates with better health and longevity. Three, many Americans desperately want to lose weight.

Only one-third of Americans boast a "normal" weight for their height. About a third are overweight but not obese; more than a third are obese. Over the past three decades, the proportion of obese adults has doubled from 15 percent to nearly 36 percent. The number of overweight children has tripled. More than 30 percent of children and adolescents are overweight or obese. "Globesity" is a word coined to reflect the worldwide epidemic of obesity.

Before we go further, we'd like to point out that body fat has benefits. It forms cell membranes, fills out the contours of your face, insulates you from the cold, and cushions your bones and organs. Excessive fat, however, especially when it's deposited in your abdomen, undermines health. This so-called visceral fat releases inflammatory chemicals and a number of proteins.

The net result of excess body weight is an increased risk for high blood pressure, atherosclerosis, heart disease, type-2 diabetes, metabolic syndrome (a clustering of risk factors for cardiovascular disease and diabetes), gallstones, gastroesophageal reflux disease (heartburn), and certain cancers. Excess fat in the throat can lead to obstructive sleep apnea, a condition marked by recurrent bouts of snoring and breath-holding, which leads to extreme daytime sleepiness and raises the risk for heart attack and stroke. Increased body weight causes low back pain and arthritis.

On the other hand, losing unhealthy body fat has benefits—even if you don't reach an "ideal" body weight. Dropping just 10 pounds (4.5 kg) can lower blood pressure, cholesterol, and triglycerides (blood fat). Changing habits that have become somewhat automatic can challenge the best of us. But it's entirely possible. Remind yourself of the changes you've willingly and successfully taken on: starting a new job, moving house, adopting a pet, getting married, or having a child. Doubtless you've already made countless transformative shifts.

Chickie-Veg Sauté

2 tablespoons (30 ml) olive oil

2 chicken breasts, skinned

½ cup (120 ml) chicken or vegetable stock, plus more as needed

2 teaspoons (2 g) herbes de Provence, divided

2 teaspoons (4 g) chopped scallion

Paprika

Freshly ground black pepper

1 cup (70 g) mushrooms, sliced

1 cup (150 g) red bell pepper, seeded and sliced

1 cup (120 g) zucchini, sliced

1 garlic clove, chopped

PREPARATION AND USE:

Pour the oil into a large skillet over medium heat and then place chicken breasts in the pan and sauté for 5 minutes on each side. Add the stock, cover the skillet, and cook over low heat for about 10 minutes until the chicken is done in the center. Remove the chicken, sprinkle with half of the herbes de Provence, scallion, and paprika and black pepper to taste, and transfer to a plate. Cover to keep warm. Add the vegetables, garlic, and rest of the herbes de Provence to the pan and sauté in the existing broth, pouring in more stock as needed to keep the vegetables moist. Cook over medium heat until tender, about 5 minutes. Add the vegetables to the chicken and serve.

YIELD: 2 servings

How it works: Dietary fat, including that found in olive oil, satisfies hunger. But a little goes a long way. Fats have more than twice the calories, gram per gram, as carbohydrates and protein. Avoid deep-fat frying. Instead, bake, broil, roast, or cook with water or broth to poach, braise, steam, or stew.

Go for Yogurt

1 cup (230 g) plain nonfat Greek yogurt
1 apple or pear, cored and chopped
¼ cup (33 g) fresh berries
Pinch of ground cinnamon

PREPARATION AND USE:
Put the yogurt into a small bowl. Add the apple and berries and mix. Top with a pinch of cinnamon. Enjoy.

YIELD: 1 serving

How it works: Adding nonfat or low-fat yogurt to the diet is associated with weight loss. Yogurt may be beneficial because it favorably alters intestinal bacteria. Fascinating lab research suggests that gut microbes influence weight. Fruit contains satisfying sweetness and fiber, which creates a sense of fullness. A study of overweight women who ate an apple or pear (versus oatmeal cookies) three times a day found that they lost an average of 2.7 pounds (1.2 kg) over twelve weeks.

Nutty Buddy To-Go

1 cup (145 g) raw almonds

1 cup (100 g) walnuts

1 teaspoon (6 g) sea salt

½ cup (80 g) dried cherries or (75 g) golden raisins

PREPARATION AND USE:

Preheat the oven to 350°F (180°C, or gas mark 4). Place the nuts on a baking sheet and toss with the salt. Spread the nuts across the sheet evenly. Roast for 30 minutes. Remove from the oven and let cool. Mix the roasted nuts with the raisins. Place in bags in small containers and keep in your purse, car, backpack, or office for snacks.

YIELD: 2 to 3 servings

How it works: Having good food on hand keeps you from snacking on junk food. Several studies indicate that people who regularly eat nuts tend to be leaner. Dried fruits, such as cherries and raisins, provide fiber and energy-maintaining carbohydrates. Nuts are satisfying and their fiber slows down their energy absorption. Walnuts are high in healthy omega-3, fatty acids, and almonds are rich in fiber, protein, calcium, and iron. However, dried fruit and nuts are relatively high in calories. Simple math dictates that adding calories to the diet results in weight gain. The goal is to substitute small amounts of nuts for less healthy snacks such as chips and candy. Note: Raw vegetables are also a good choice because they are relatively low in calories but high in fiber. Instead of fruit, pack snackable vegetables, such as baby carrots, sugar snap peas, and grape tomatoes.

Lemongrass Green Tea

½ cup (33 g) chopped fresh lemongrass

3 cups (710 ml) water, divided

2 teaspoons (4 g) loose green tea

Stevia

PREPARATION AND USE:

Trim the tough bottoms of the lemongrass stalks by 2 to 6 inches (5 to 15 cm). Cut the lemongrass tops into ½-inch (1.3 cm) chunks to fill ½ cup (33 g). Set aside. Bring 2 cups (475 ml) of water to a boil in a saucepan and lower the heat to a simmer. Add the lemongrass and stevia to taste, stirring to dissolve. Cover and simmer for 20 minutes. Add the green tea. Remove from the heat and steep 3 minutes. In a blender, blend the mixture so that the lemongrass pieces are finely minced. Strain the tea into a pitcher, removing the tea and lemongrass particles. Discard these. You should have a little more than 1 cup (235 ml) left. Add remaining cup (235 ml) of water. Stir in additional stevia to taste. If you prefer your drinks cold, serve over ice.

YIELD: 2 servings

How it works: Green tea contains caffeine (though not as much as coffee) and substances called green tea polyphenols. Some, but not all, studies indicate that concentrated green tea extracts that concentrate the polyphenols lead to weight loss. Lemongrass (*Cymbopogon citratus*), which is native to India and Southeast Asia, creates a zingy taste. Stevia-based sweeteners are made from extracts of the leaves of Stevia rebaudiana, a South American plant used for centuries as a sweetener. Gram for gram, it's much sweeter than table sugar and contains no calories.

Step It Up

See the Lifestyle Tips throughout the book for more ideas on how to move.

You

Comfortable workout clothes

A pair of athletic shoes

PREPARATION AND USE:

For 60 minutes every day, walk, jog, ride the elliptical trainer, swim, play tennis, or do a combination of these activities.

YIELD: 1 daily session (Work up to 90 minutes each day for weight loss.)

How it works: Sedentary lifestyles foster weight gain. Being more physically active directly burns calories. Exercises that build muscle lead to higher metabolic rate at rest. Muscle consumes more calories than body fat. Studies show that regular exercise can overturn genetic predispositions to be overweight. Experts recommend 60 minutes a day of moderate-intensity exercise to prevent weight gain and 90 minutes to lose weight. It's perfectly fine to exercise in 10-minute chunks.

Exercise has the added benefits of increasing total body function, boosting your self-esteem, and helping you sleep better at night. To shed excess weight, calories expended in exercise need to outnumber the calories in your diet. If exercise piques your appetite, satisfy your hunger with fruits vegetables, fish, lean meats, and nuts.